MARY TAKAKI- A

The Inside-Outside

Diet

Lose the Mental Weight

Lose the Emotional Weight

Lose the PHYSICAL Weight

* Permanently *

by Mark E. Laursen MD, ABHM

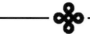

www.NaturalBodyHealth.com

888-NATRLMD (888-628-7563)

866-XTRALIFE (866-987-2543)

This book is dedicated to my sisters Marilyn Jan, Becky Marie, Belinda Ann and Lisa Kay.

This book is also dedicated to my parents Barbara Jean and Larry Eugene Laursen.

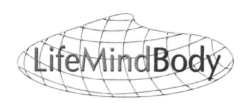

www.LifeMindBody.net

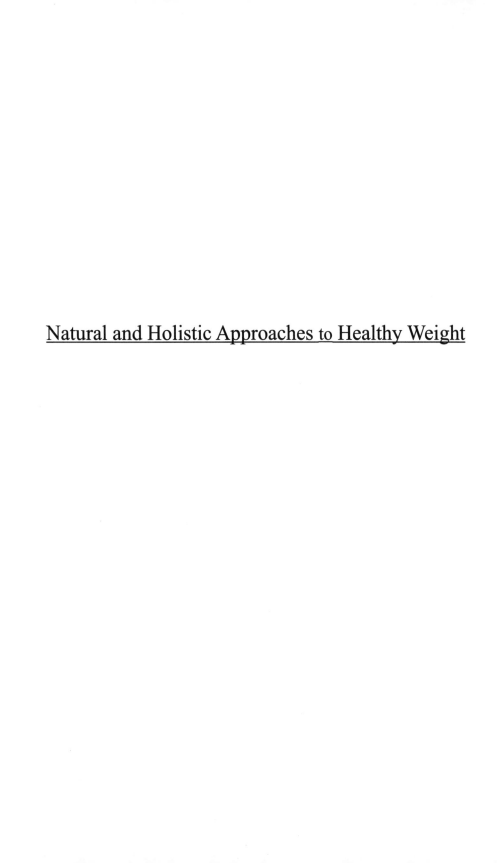

Natural and Holistic Approaches to Healthy Weight

I would like to thank my wife Kathy for her suggestions and constant support in the development of this book.

I would like to acknowledge the edit of this book by Ms. Constance DeSwaan.

Layout by Clyde Bernederskitter.

Think of a new way to live.

Forward

The purpose of this book is much more than helping you simply lose weight, but to help you holistically acquire the knowledge and inner changes that will *require* your body to be automatically healthier. More than the most complete weight loss/diet book ever written, it is a therapeutic guide to know thyself, love thyself, change thyself and revitalize your life.

The Inside-Outside Diet will reveal all the holistic methods you can use to improve your weight using "Outside" approaches of understanding better food, supplements, herbs, exercise and lifestyle choices. The Inside-Outside Diet will also show you how to neutralize binging, addictive eating and compulsive overeating that you previously have not had the willpower to alter – the "Inside" techniques of change.

Altering your energy, your thoughts and emotions to make them natural and healthy can decrease your cravings. Correct foods and supplements create mood stability. Your body will naturally not want to eat as much, and you will lose weight just as naturally. This book will help to bring out the inner natural you that currently lives behind a wall of discontent and misplaced drives.

Most of why we overeat is based on our state of energy. Need your energy increased and feel more pleasure? In your past you would have turned to sugary foods, soda pop, coffee and stimulants. Need your energy decreased and stress taken away? You would have eaten chocolate, fatty foods and those high in carbohydrates. *Why* you have energy needs that go up and down and drive you to remedy them with food is crucial to know.

You do just about everything based on energy and how you feel. Why your energy cycles up and down is not just because of your food intake, it's about your decisions and beliefs that create these energy drives. Understand these energy clues, optimize your food and nutrient choices and use the techniques to change your emotions and drives, then you will be a different person--the one we've been waiting for all along.

We are at a time in history that our culture has developed four unrecognized situations that greatly affect our health. Unfortunately, modern science and medicine have overlooked them.

ONE: Our culture has developed such a stressful nature related to lifestyles and financial survival that this upsets the inner neurohormonal balance of mankind's happiness–all of which cause increasing psychological and physical illness.

TWO: For the first time in recent history, the physical requirements for work and survival have become minimal for the majority of the population. Our bodies, being biochemical and bio-physical organisms, have incurred biochemical changes from this lack of use that result in increased susceptibility to illness and disease, including obesity.

As a very important example of this for diabetics and overweight people, consider the dynamic relationship of sugar, fat and muscles in the body. 75% of the sugar in the body and blood goes to use by the muscles *normally*. When you stop using your muscles and have less muscle mass in general (lean body mass), your muscle cells become less "needy" and your sugar has to go somewhere else instead. Insulin is the hormone produced by the pancreas that lowers the sugar content of the body. If your muscles can't use the sugar then the body converts it with insulin to fat.

When you are not *using* your muscles then you are backing up to a certain extent the normal flow and use of sugar in the blood. Or when you over-supply the body with excessive eaten sugar and to a degree starchy carbohydrates, the sugar is converted to fat all over the body including your arteries. Insulin levels go up, fat levels go up, blood pressure goes up wreaking havoc on the muscles, blood vessels and body. When you lose weight and obtain a healthier lean body mass, many people cure diabetes and normalize their blood pressure. It is possible to lose weight and reset your neuro-hormonal metabolism. You return your insulin-fat relationship to normal. Overeating is an insulin problem on the physical plane.

THREE: Our food supply, both manufactured and produced, has become nutrient deficient, leading to increased susceptibility to illness. Essential nutrients are ones the body must consume because the body can't manufacture them. Trace minerals are examples of essential nutrients often missing in modern food. The body will malfunction without them.

FOUR: Foreign, unnatural, toxic food and poor eating habits have become ingrained in the food business, causing poor health and disease such as cancers and chronic illness. The business world of food companies, retail suppliers and financial interests have often deliberately created a culture of fear, emotional manipulation and false food/happiness relationships that have become indoctrinated into the cultures of many "modern countries," greatly contributing to the cultural promotion of ill health, obesity and other personal and social diseases.

Motivation, knowledge, proper food and supplements are what you need to achieve healthy weight loss. Knowledge is the essence of what *The Inside Outside Diet* provides. This information will also enable you to choose the right foods and supplements that will assist you in your health quest. Motivation can be helped also, but that still must ultimately come from you.

The Inside-Outside Diet provides powerful concepts and tools that will compel healthier life, and it starts with you!

Hummingbirds

Hummingbirds don't fly
       They move by Beaute.'
I've never seen their wings.
       I feel sorry for them to have two feet and no wings.
Surely they are handicapped.

Why do they keep staring into those flowers?
       Do they see their reflection
Or is it their shadow (they are trying to see)?
       Trying to see if they have wings.
They must know they're handicapped.

I feel sorry for them
       to have no hands or wings.
Why don't they walk?
       I saw one sitting on a branch one day.
I do not think it could find any Beaute'.
       I was sad.

I wanted to eat the bird.
       It flew away.
Maybe that's what happened to hummingbirds,
       Someone ate their wings.
I would keep on flying to Beaute' too,
       If I had wings.

I have flowers, but they are too low for me.
       And I can't fly, I have no wings.
So what's the use of trying.
       What is Beaute'?
What is Beaute' anyway?

Clyde B. 22-11-90

Contents

Part III
Outside-In Changes for Weight Loss

Part IV
Special Situations and Conditions

"It feels good to be light again"

Too much eating of wrong foods and the harm they cause is difficult to research in modern science labs. This is due to the prolonged time of testing required for investigation of chronic and subtle food irritants and allergies.

Preface

Okay, you have excess weight. Lurking somewhere beneath your lifestyle that's just not working for you anymore on too many levels lies a desire to be more healthy and definitely more fit. It means: To be able to cross your legs or wear clothes that are more form fitting and less a matter of covering up. To be self-approving of your body, to be happier, to live longer, to never buy larger-size clothes again? If all this happened, you think, you could experience and enjoy life again, look into a mirror and feel good about yourself, be empowered and have self-mastery over your life! You probably believe that having all this hinges on finding a better weight-loss diet-- the miracle fix!

The truth is that 80 million Americans diet each year, and 95 % of them gain all the weight back within five years. Why? The reason is simple: 95 % of those dieters never correct the original reason for their being overweight in the first place. But it can be done. Those 95 percent can change and so can you when you understand that <u>you have to lose the "mental weight" to lose the "emotional weight" to then *permanently* lose the physical weight.</u>

So many people sincerely want to lose weight--I see this every day in my practice--yet they haven't succeeded because they are paying attention to all the wrong things. Scientific information on nutrition, diet styles and medical discoveries about how our bodies work pour forth, putting attention onto foods, the glycemic index, low carbs, and on and on. Still, people find it difficult to permanently keep weight off, even if they temporarily achieve some weight loss. <u>Why?</u> The fundamental answer is that people have not found within themselves the true origin of how they became overweight. All that science and medical testing have been able to do is shed a small amount of light on the physical process of gaining weight. Typically modern Americans, we have looked for the causes of our problems as being outside of us, and just as counterproductive, we seek solutions to our problems from the outside, too.

So where is the answer? It lies where science and medicine fear to tread, what science and medicine know the least about--what's in your very mind, the mind that has directed your life, in the emotions that have created your lifestyle and body, and in the very culture that society has created. Society is out of step with health in general, and too many people default into that unhealthy way of thinking and wind up out of shape and overweight. Being overweight has to have an impact on the rest of your life. But you have a choice -- a path to travel to health or decline.

Give yourself a break. Simplify. Deal with the fundamentals of *why* you are overweight and you won't ever be overweight again, nor out of shape, nor probably even in ill health whatsoever.

The reason people can't lose weight is because they don't *feel* they can, or they don't have the willpower and they haven't understood the exact mechanism that led them to become overweight in the first place. Other feelings at times compel people to overeat. Their willpower can't overcome their feelings at the moment their drive to eat becomes too strong. So you know, reasonably, you shouldn't have a second supersize chocolate bar, but you give in anyway. You can change bad choices like this, however, so it will make a difference next time. You will have to use the holistic techniques of the Inside-Outside Diet to alter your habits and go counter to your culture that says, sure, chocolate and coffee are the right choices to satisfy some drives. You will have to create new healthy, positive compelling memories to form new drives that replace the old negative ones of the past.

My goal for you is to get you healthy and happy again. I'll do this by showing you that the answers lay inside your mind and emotions, which you have created. This book is about the natural, Outside-In *and* Inside-Out ways to improve your health and weight. These Outside-In actions are those you make in your environment such as choosing the right foods, electrolytes, amino acids, herbs and exercise that will improve your weight and energy–plus they might save you from diabetes or metabolic syndrome. But most importantly, I'll guide you toward succeeding with the ultimate Inside-Out methods to permanently end excess weight in your life. These Inside forces are ones you **must** change to eliminate excess weight and maintain it. **First, you must take responsibility for your health and your weight to change them.**

You can take Outside-In steps to heal, but you can only cure yourself from the Inside-Out. I'll help you by providing plans, goals and techniques that empower you to accomplish this.

Many of these techniques are located in my premier "foundation of health" book, *Start Living Stop Dying - 10 Steps to Natural Health,* which you should read and understand prior to implementing *The Inside Outside Diet.* I'll greatly expand on why these techniques are important here. Use these techniques to change yourself and you will regain a healthy self-concept, improved attitude, a sense of security and well-being which manifest in healthier life choices.

The Inside-Outside Diet will provide you with everything necessary to achieve healthy permanent weight loss. In less than a year, you will discover and change your desire to overeat. This book will change your life and provide you with a solid foundation for your perfect body, inside and out.

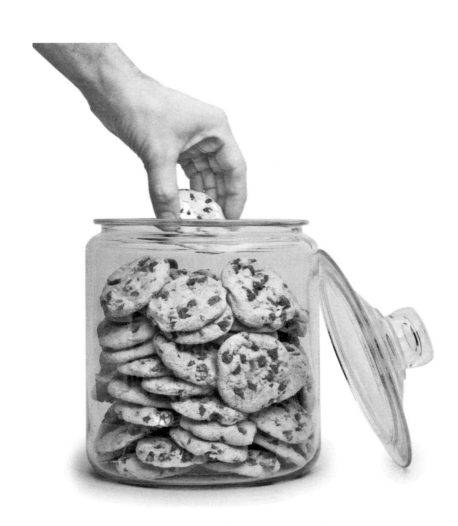

Part I:

The Core: Getting Started on the Inside-Outside Journey to Healthy Weight

Chapter One

Inside the Cookie Jar

-Who stole the cookie from the cookie jar? Who me? Yes you! Couldn't be! Then who?

-Mama stole the cookie from the cookie jar! Who me? Yes you. Couldn't be! Then who?

-Daddy stole the cookie from the cookie jar! Who me? Yes you! Couldn't be! Then who?

For a long time no one has taken responsibility for the growing obesity epidemic in the United States. Of course, it's more than raids on the cookie jar--it's family and social history, cultural habits, wrong foods, survival stress, manipulative manufacturing and vending practices, poor eating habits, even poorer nutritional information and the great emotional component: the comfort of food. It all ends with problems of being overweight at any possible level and age.

We know the number of people who are overweight is exploding according to various statistics. Our children are especially overweight, with 25 million of them in the United States. Obesity may be the highest factor associated with all illnesses and poor quality of life. Excess weight is associated with high blood pressure, diabetes, arthritic joint pains, cardiac problems, back pain and atherosclerosis, which is the usual ultimate cause of everyone's physical demise. Being overweight is also associated with increasing likelihoods of getting breast cancer, prostate cancer, colon cancer, stroke, depression, gallstones, GERD, varicose veins and the list will likely go on and on. If you have already dealt with these illnesses, they can serve as motivations to regain a healthy weight now as many of these conditions are reversible with normal weight. Correcting your weight back to a healthy state has ramifications for anyone seeking to improve their quality of life. The medical concerns affect you and me.

Obesity is now considered a disease of its own. We've also been told that obesity is climbing from second to first place as the leading contributor to death. According to the conservative Journal of the American Medical Association, 67% of the American population is overweight and 16% of our kids. At the rate we are losing good health, in 10 years, 95 percent of the population may be overweight whose future medical treatment could very well bankrupt the national healthcare system.

There are medical reasons for being overweight for which you should see a doctor. Besides hypothyroidism, which can be caused by a deficiency of iodine in your body or Hashimoto's disease, there are polycystic ovarian disease, Cushing's disease and adrenal dysfunction. All of these are hormonal disorders associated with weight gain but do not have a true cause identified in traditional medicine. Alternative therapies including herbs and nutrients may be useful for these situations, in addition to the standard medical approaches for dealing with their symptoms.

Hashimoto's thyroiditis is an autoimmune condition where the body's immune system attacks the thyroid gland itself and is associated with hypothyroidism. There is no accepted standard medical treatment for this condition at this time other than thyroid replacement. However, some alternative doctors have reported improvements with these patients taking omega 3 fatty acids, selenium 100-200 mcg a day for 6 months, vitamin D, glutathione and vitamin E. If you have this condition, I would suggest you eat hypoallergenic foods, particularly not having gluten or cow dairy. (Paleolithic diet). Consult your doctor for potential treatment options.

Polycystic ovarian disease is a condition involving increased androgen synthesis by the body. Diet and exercise are commonly recommended along with the prescribed drug metformin. Cushing syndrome is a rare condition involving sustained high cortisol levels. Adrenal dysfunction or exhaustion is a condition of low cortisol and can be treated with steroids. Herbal therapies exist for both of these conditions.

You are also at risk of developing metabolic syndrome (syndrome X) and diabetes if you are overweight. 50 million Americans will develop metabolic syndrome according to recent studies and they will begin to show signs of hypertension, elevated lipid levels and elevated insulin levels with insulin resistance. Your doctor can order laboratory tests to check on all of these conditions. Having other physical ailments or co-morbidities may also play a role in your ability to exercise.

The myth that anyone has a "slow metabolism" is partially true. You can have thyroid dysfunction causing a slower metabolism but your basal metabolic rate can also increase when you add muscle mass to your frame. It is in part why exercise and in particular, strength training, is so important for revving up metabolism and keeping weight down. The more muscle you have, the higher resting metabolic rate you will generate and the more calories you will burn every day, whether you exercise or not. For every one pound of lean muscle mass you can add to your body, you will automatically burn 60 more calories each day.

What most people look at for being overweight is the BMI, which is your body mass index (greater than 30 = obesity), which is a calculation of weight over height. Your waist circumference is also a rough guide to determine if you are overweight, but a more accurate measure is what percentage of body fat is excess weight. While the mirror will reveal if you are obviously overweight, there are a large number of people who look normal but are actually "over fat" with a body fat percentage of 25- 45 percent. They are at risk of developing metabolic syndrome which is a "pre-diabetic" condition.

What's more, for those stepping on the scale, the actual ideal body weight currently recommended today is still too heavy, that is, about five percent over what is truly ideal body weight. The best body for most people is slender, given some expected genetic variance among cultures and individuals. That's about 9-12 percent body fat for adult men and 12-16 percent body fat for adult women. However, how you feel may be the most important motivating determinant of your health–so how are you feeling?

In the dark days of dealing solely with weight loss as the problem, doctors would say that overweight people simply lacked the willpower to lose weight--or were lazy. Modern day doctors specializing in the treatment of weight loss, armed with many more scientific studies, would say overweight people do not lack willpower. Nor are they lazy. Rather, they're more likely to attribute excess weight to hormonal imbalance, ghrelin and leptin alterations, abnormal fat cells and high glycemic foods swinging blood sugar levels up and down, greatly influencing and driving uncontrollable feelings of hunger to the brain.

The truth is that both theories are correct. Holistically speaking, physical, emotional and mental conditions are connected. Willpower, beliefs, emotional drives and the body are all in communication through energy. Food is more than calories, it contains information, energy and substance that relates to neuro-hormones, emotions and thoughts.

Why are you overweight? This is an important question.

Where do the drives to eat more than we need come from? For many people, overeating is a byproduct of a frustrating pattern of life. Most overweight people who wish to lose weight can't stop eating and can't maintain an exercise program. They do not have the willpower to stop binging, indulging in cravings, overeating and eating wrong kinds of food. This drive to overeat has a deep emotional underpinning and origin--it doesn't exist on its own. To control hunger, you have to satisfy mental boredom, emotional anxiety and physical need.

Where overweight people shortchange themselves is by believing that they cannot consciously change their willpower, beliefs, drives, emotions, feelings and convictions to create lasting health and weight change. Of course, you can!

Diets never touch the heart of why you become overweight

The truth about why you're overweight isn't one answer--there are many aspects to adding on excess weight as there are getting back to a healthy weight. But, you can break through and figure it out with this help. You can work on all aspects of getting healthy, including food choices, exercise and lifestyle or work on them one at a time. You absolutely must change certain emotions and beliefs that hold you back if you want to permanently change your weight. This means you have to change you – and I'll show you how.

Your physical body reveals the true inner reality of the undermining beliefs and emotions that you generate as you interact in the world around you. However, you have control over most of how you respond and how you think. Everything is doable or possible to the person whose mind reflects correct thoughts and awareness, backed by the conviction of willpower and emotion behind it. So, if you're overweight, there are four key reasons in the primary chain of how that happens:

●People who are overweight, overeat.

●People overeat because they misuse or misinterpret true hunger.

Appetite, or hunger, is a desire to alter energy, to affect a change in your sense of well-being.

The primary causes of overeating in the United States are due to two powerful psychological and emotional motivations arising from within:

●People overeat because of a need for pleasure and to escape feeling bored. Thus, we raise our energy when it feels too low.

●People overeat as a means to relieve, dump or balance emotional stress and anxiety. We lower our excess energy when it is too high. We do all this eating and changing of energy to *feel* better.

What are your chances for losing poundage and finally getting your body in balance if you only focus your mind on food diets? Very few! You could diet all year long or over your entire lifetime and you'll never deal with or remedy the emotional causes for overeating by merely changing your food regimen. **In fact, being on a diet will actually increase thoughts and preoccupation with food; and your weight will increase and return--*but you know that!***

First, let's take a look at how we got to where we are today in the passing of the diets that have paved the way to understanding weight loss.

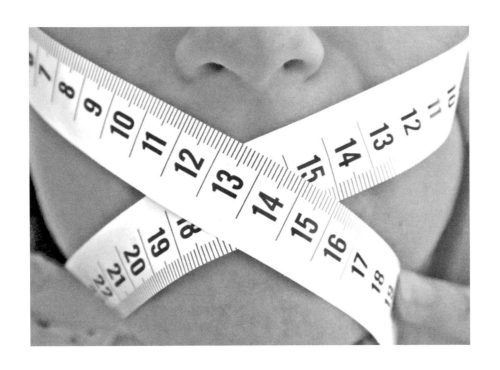

95 % of All Diets

Lead to Increased

Eating

Chapter Two

Fads, Trends and
Other Unhealthy Diet Choices

Yes, even popular diets can cause havoc with your system. You may lose weight initially with them, but the long-term results are more far-reaching: they're not only useless, but potential health hazards.

Why Diets Don't Work

Patients always ask why diets don't work, since they are set up for weight loss. Or, are they? The problem is that almost all diets focus on food and the outside factors and inherently fail you! The old thinking that the problem of gaining weight was something outside of you (food) and the solution was also outside of you (better food) has proven totally wrong! Diets tend to *increase* thinking of food and result in **"rebound eating"** where you later indulge in everything you thought about eating earlier but didn't, thus, gaining back even more weight than when you started. Diets prime the mind to eat. The 95 percent of people who lose weight and then regain weight is not because of the food, but due to your mind's *focus on food*.

Your mind is like a computer--once you load it with thoughts and ideas, it runs efficiently, manifesting all the "data" you inserted. Tell yourself you can eat chocolate and your mind will think about it. Tell your mind you cannot eat chocolate and your mind will run that idea also. *Both* thoughts magnify your preoccupation with food.

Believe you cannot live without soda pop, or, that eating less equals a deprivation you cannot deal with for more than two weeks, (the number of days for most fast weight-loss diets) then you cannot do anything but gain weight back. When you leave the diet, run for the candy or snacks and gain back more weight, your confidence and self-esteem diminish. These are the very traits you need to *strengthen* your belief system that says you *can* change yourself. Clearly, dieting can be more harmful than helpful over the long term.

Many diets are also unnatural and dangerous. They include unnatural foods and artificial additives such as artificial sweeteners, which have no calories, but are potentially more chemically bad for your system! Diet drinks have some of the highest AGE's which stand for "Advanced Glycosylated End-products" which are some of the highest carcinogenic products you can ingest, which diet sodas contain, for example.

Which leads me to another question patients ask: What kind of diet, then, should I follow? My answer is that **the best diet is a "non-diet!"** A non-diet does not focus on food or create an obsession for it. Rather, it includes lifestyle shifts as well as techniques to lose the mental and emotional weight that have gotten in the way of maintaining a healthy body weight. You can use self-discipline for a while so that you believe your diet really helps you achieve weight loss, but if your energy is amiss, you are pleasure deprived, depressed, overwhelmed, overstressed or overworked, these true inner feelings will seek relief and balance, even if that means eating for pleasure or eating for tension release.

The need for joy that's missing in your life eventually wrecks any self-discipline you may have about sticking to your food diet. Add further worries about your life, job, money or relationships and it will increase tension and lead to yet more relief eating or binging. You must have **non-eating joys** in your life plan and you must personally allow yourself to have joy. Many people have difficulty allowing themselves to feel joy.

There will always be a mental thought process you maintain and a resulting emotional energy you have created, collected or stored in your body that has caused your illness or obesity. Give yourself the benefit of discovering it, facing and letting it go! It's the internal drives that must be self-examined and then altered to achieve lasting change.

The food-emphasizing diets (which all diets are that I know of to date) do just that--they emphasize food and are totally wrong to lose weight. You need to emphasize health and leanness with right thoughts and emotions to build your mind up with these concepts. You must walk, run or do some form of exercise like yoga; change your stress level, lifestyle and balance your energy. Return your body to youthful functioning, peaceful energy and vitality. Optionally, you can fast to strengthen emotional awareness and lose weight. *You have an ability to hit your reset button of life whenever you contemplate or meditate, rejuvenate your emotions or fast.*

Education *about* food is important however and I will discuss in greater detail more of this topic later in the section of "Holistic Nutrition." For now, simply follow what is natural when choosing foods from the grocery store or restaurant. Eat seasonally and stop eating all foods sometime, by which I mean give yourself a break from eating any one food continuously. (The same safe philosophy also applies to supplements – you should come off them every so often to return to normal body function.) **So what's wrong with your diet? Are you ready to get beyond your diet dilemma?**

The following diets you may have heard about or tried and are summarized as follows. They have all contributed to our greater understanding of healthy living. Along with contributions, all of these diets have major shortcomings, particularly in that they don't show you how to deal with your original emotional problems or beliefs that led you to gain weight. They don't provide techniques for you to have permanent change and therefore permanent weight loss. Many of these diets prescribe foods that often are unnatural and toxic. Ninety-five percent of the health food bars or health foods I've examined contain nitrates, nitrites, sulfates, hydrogenated oils, salt and artificial flavorings that damage your body – that's how wrong the health food industry has been. All wrong energy and information to send into your body.

*The **Low-Carb Diet** has been the phenomenon of the last 10 years starting with Dr. Atkins' diet plan. No diet has ever had such a far reaching effect as the **Atkins Diet**. While criticized for bucking the medical establishment, his philosophy was based on correct body physiology of fat production and destruction. Originally, Dr. Atkins' plan was quite unnatural for most people's body evolution and inherently required a substituted high-fat and high-protein diet. If you weren't eating carbohydrates, you had to be eating a lot of fat and protein.

Dr. Atkins recommended not eating sugars and carbohydrates while allowing you to eat all the protein and fats you want. All that you want! This simplicity really appealed to the general public. When people think of diets, they think of something that's hard, something that they cannot wait to stop doing. But the Atkins Diet originally said eat all that you want: have a steak and heap on a whipped cream topping. On the surface, that seems easy, if not too good to be true. Sure, most cardiologists will tell me that I should eat meat in moderation, but it's hard for someone who's losing weight to stop the diet. Nowadays, the diet says to limit fat to 20 percent of your calories so it has come to a more moderate stance. That is good, but it changes what the diet was originally about, and people will often ignore that change.

At one time, so many people were on this diet that the price of meat and dairy soared. Scientists are actually trying to genetically engineer protein foods to taste like carbohydrates. How many generations will it take to find the dangers in these new genetically modified and unnatural foods?

The Atkins Diet does work when strictly done, causes weight loss, taking advantage of biophysical pathways of metabolism in the body. Our bodies convert carbohydrates into sugars, and we can only burn these sugars so fast, thus excess sugars get stored in the form of fat. If you don't eat carbohydrates in moderation or you eat a lot of refined sugar, you will put on fat. And if you stop eating carbohydrates, your body will go into reverse, burning fat for energy.

The real problem in modern society that the Atkins Diet addressed is the massive amount of sugar that we consume. But the complex carbohydrates can still be very good for people. It's the sugar that people really need to eliminate to improve their health. Every cola, orange juice, milk and sugar drink needs to be removed from your refrigerator because they never were healthy products to consume.

Every cola, orange juice, milk and sugar drink needs to be removed from your refrigerator

Dangers of ill health are all potential consequences of following any low-carb, high-protein, high-fat diet for long periods of time. Over the short term of probably less than six months, the body handles most temporary food changes quite well and may actually improve some of your blood lipid markers that doctors currently monitor. Providing you have a decent body health prior to this diet and do not have underlying kidney disease or liver problems, you may initially benefit from the low-carb diet as far as losing weight goes. Over the long term however, high protein diets may damage your kidneys, and fat may stress or damage multiple body systems from your liver to your gallbladder to your very arteries themselves in the form of atherosclerosis. The threat of atherosclerosis is the primary concern of high-fat diets. Still, there is evidence that supplementing with at least three grams of fish oil a day may protect you from progressing to atherosclerosis no matter what your lipid levels.

People who go on a low-carb diet are using "outside" means to reduce weight and are, at best, obtaining temporary results, but never a cure. By following it, you're trading one physical problem (overweight) for others to come, including potential kidney problems and atherosclerosis, while never curing the original cause of why you're overweight. Kidney malfunctioning in general is increasing in the world due to diabetes, drugs and foreign compounds taken into the body.

High protein can overload the kidney with ammonia and urea compounds and, in fact, can be used to measure the kidney function by whether these two compounds are backed up in the body from a kidney unable to filter them out properly. Protein makes urea, ammonia and creatinine in the body, which have to be excreted.

The high protein diet has been said also to stress the liver and adrenal glands leading to poor health and progressively less energy. The higher protein absorption may also lead to direct increased allergenicity. People who work out think that they need to eat more protein to make more muscle and so they eat cans of tuna to bulk up. However two of the most muscled and strongest animals, gorillas and bulls, are vegetarians. Even human infants during the biggest growth cycle of their lives consume breast milk which is less than two percent protein.

Protein has low caloric value and tends to get metabolized into energy molecules or other useful amino acid groups for muscles and neuro-peptides. Fats eaten usually get broken down into energy molecules and are less likely to get stored as fat. It would seem the opposite but that's how the body works biochemically in short.

The relatively higher fat consumption in a high-protein/high-fat/low-carb diet means you're taking in a lot of calories that still must somehow be burned up. High-fat consumption has traced to high levels of lipoprotein and fat in your blood which have been linked with cardiovascular and blood vessel problems that result in heart attacks and strokes. Since these two are still big killers, a high fat diet only sounds risky to me.

There is overwhelming evidence that high-fat diets lead to heart disease, cancer of the colon, prostate, breast and more. These unusually high fat diets also relate to diabetes, hypertension and gallbladder problems. With long term high fat, high protein and probably high foreign chemical intake, too, you may be hurting your body.

Even if you can eat all the meat that you want, potatoes and pizza sure are nice to eat sometimes and we get to missing them like old friends. Because we never got to the heart of our food issues while on this diet, sooner or later, there's a high-carb binge coming on full force–and guilt and remorse to follow it.

Still we must give Dr. Atkins credit for letting the world know how ketosis burns fat and correctly turning people away from damaging sugar consumption. Remember that heart disease and cancer are lowest with vegetarian diets which are pretty much the opposite of Atkins. If you ever get to see a gorilla or bull in the wild (not to mention race horses!) you will see a very vital, fit, muscled and vegetarian animal, healthier than most people.

*Most of the other popular diets of today are low-carb or low-carb/high-protein variations of the Atkins Diet. The **South Beach Diet** emphasizes eliminating carbohydrates with high absorption (high glycemic index) or eating them with other foods that slow down their absorption. This effect is valid but falls far short of the goal of permanent weight loss. Now the literature of the diet advertises that you can eat all foods, without exercise, and it doesn't matter if you're depressed--it works for binge eating and no willpower is necessary. For me, that immediately cuts the credibility of the diet, trying to appeal to those who want something for nothing.

At best, the outside factors of food and weight are all that the

South Beach Diet considers. The diet says you can have chocolate and caffeine which many people will love to hear and as long as people are more interested in what they want to hear than the truth, this diet will have a market. This diet recommends unnatural canola oil which I consider harmful, and peanut oil which is allergenic for many people. Although these diets may temporarily work, true health will come from more individualized factors such as finding your own best foods and getting to the core beliefs and your lifestyle that cause you to overeat.

*The **Pritikin Diet**, started in the 1950's, but which took off in the 1970's, introduced useful concepts for healthy living and the fundamentals for the following half century of diets. Good for cardiac patients and anyone else, it reduced the intake of meat and fat while increasing fiber. It emphasized watching calories to lose weight, and it also included exercise for weight control. However, Dr. Pritikin did not know to include important fats such as omega 3 essential fatty acids, and like most diets, this one did not address the mental and emotional issues related to health and obesity.

With the Pritikin Diet came a giant trend in our approach to food. The popular interest in calorie counting became a good way to market commercial products like Special K and Diet Pepsi in the 1960's. Companies have since profited from a series of unnatural and questionably safe artificial sweeteners, synthesized to be sweet without the calories. And diets became an important part of our culture. Much like the fashions that we put on our bodies, these trendy combinations of new foods to put in our bodies sold magazines and books right off the racks. Sadly, as consumers we had decided to let "experts" give us lists of foods to eat instead of learning from our own sensations what foods really felt good for our own bodies.

*Published in 1987, the **Dean Ornish Diet** ushered in the era of "scientifically based" diets. Emphasizing more low-calorie foods to lose weight, it was also an ultra low-fat diet. Less fat has been linked to fewer vascular problems, fewer cardiac events and less cancer, so it was extremely good for people with cardiac and cancer concerns, which is almost everyone. These are still the two most likely health problems to end your life. Still recommended today, the diet now emphasizes yoga and meditation, making stress relief a very real component of this methodology.

However, not eating fat can be difficult for some people and the detrimental effects of eating any sugar is probably one of the worst food trends that remain with us today. With our foods, the science of one year keeps getting reversed by another year of scientific studies and product advertisements. The truth about eating fats and carbohydrates will probably come to rest somewhere in the middle, or moderation. And each of us will have our own individual biochemistry of truth to consider.

*Based on the finding that people living around the Mediterranean had less heart disease, the **Mediterranean Diet** recommends a diverse selection of foods, including vegetables, legumes, fruits, whole grains, beans, nuts and seeds. People in that region eat polenta, pasta, olives, potatoes, bulgur and rice. This diet is more about an eating practice and a lifestyle than the foods themselves. Mediterraneans had more physical activity so the Mediterranean diet says you should too.

Mediterraneans ate much of their foods raw or minimally processed with a lot of olive oil. Meals had little dairy and they preferred cheese over milk. They ate bread, but without butter or margarine. Mediterraneans did not eat much meat and they preferred fish over other meats. They did drink wine, did eat ripe fruit, and enjoyed the beneficial effects of bacterial cultures in yogurt. All in all, this sounds like a pretty healthy diet, even if we can't all have the stress-reducing effects of living by the Aegean. In fact, this diet does not give any consideration at all to the emotional and mental aspects to health.

Phil McGraw's Diet plan came along and addressed

superficially the psychology of being overweight, asking people to look at their mental reasons for why they eat too much. This was a refreshing step in the right direction, but to affect permanent change, we have to explore this more deeply and find the original causes behind the surface reasons that he asks people to examine and correct. He suggests that people throw away negative thoughts, but doesn't say how to stop them from originating. This lack of completeness leads to temporary weight loss without the self-correction that can make it complete. Nonetheless, although it is not a totally self-empowering approach, this aspect is clearly a step in the right direction.

Dr. McGraw, a psychologist, uses conventional medical approaches to the food aspects of weight loss, and his diet bars are available at many stores. They contain many ingredients that I consider harmful: sugar, cocoa, palm kernel oil, artificial flavors, synthetic vitamin E and more. The diet bars also contain allergenic foods such as peanuts which cause problems for many people. These types of products are used because of their cheapness which tells you a lot about the framework of the plan. Health food should be healthy and natural. I gave one of the bars to my dog and he wouldn't eat it. Dr. McGraw also has told people on his show that he "will make them lose weight," but the reality is that everyone must accomplish this themselves through their own will for it to be permanent. It is the individual psyche that must work on itself to accomplish a total and, therefore, spiritual change, and this deep approach is lacking in this superficial and toxic food plan.

*The **Diet Cure** takes an extremely scientific approach to weight loss and mood swings by using amino acid therapy to affect our neurotransmitters and therefore our mood. Using amino acids instead of anti-depressants is a much more natural approach to combating depression. These amino acids also improve sleep. The goal of leveling out extreme moods is important to controlling overeating. However, combating depression and obesity on a chemical/scientific basis only, without dealing with the invisible mental and emotional orbs, will limit permanent success. Thoughts, though invisible, are as real as a rock and must be dealt with in that certainty.

*The **Zone Diet** pairs sweets with protein to offset and maintain a moderate sugar level in your body. This can dampen momentary blood sugar levels and reduce lows and highs in mood. It does this by slowing sugar absorption from foods and keeping sugar spikes from happening. By using the glycemic index to control the glycemic load levels of foods, the Zone diet works much like the South Beach Diet, but it addresses a very limited aspect of weight impact and total health, and does not address mental/emotional issues.

*The **New Glucose Revolution Diet** centers more specifically around the glycemic index, a ranking of foods as to how they affect blood glucose levels. Certain foods have a quick sugar response, but their overall amount of sugar effect is very low. Glycemic "load" factors this into a food's sugar effect by considering the total amount a food has combined with its glycemic index. Studying tables of glycemic indexes may be particularly interesting to more scientifically-minded people who might be surprised by the relative differences in food glycemic indexes and their glycemic load. Keeping sugar levels on an even keel can help maintain a more stable mood. However, this is only one piece of your right foods puzzle. And once again, your emotional issues play a key role in your overall health.

Planned Meal Diets

***Weight Watchers, NutriSystem, Medifast** and the **Slimfast Diet** are based upon calorie reduction with tailored meals or "slimming" drinks. Weight Watchers has many years and millions of inches of weight loss under its belt. It does work with its members' diets, but the Weight Watchers web site actually says very little about their food. Most of their emphasis is on weekly meetings and personal support to enforce your calorie restriction. Dependence upon others is reinforced with Weight Watchers while the constant food emphasis actually increases thoughts about food that will eventually manifest itself at some point by increased eating.

Diet groups rely on a planned-meal schedule, usually selling the somewhat unnatural food produced by their company. These groups remain popular and would be better if they did not have unnatural food ingredients. People can do well with these programs for a while since the company's pitch and "motivational" sessions get their minds committed and structured--they spend a lot of time actively planning all their weight loss meals. Since people like food, people tend to like "diet" plans where they get to think more about food.

But these diets never touch the heart of *why* you become overweight in the first place, and can actually result in setbacks if you don't deal with your original reasons for emotional overeating. That is, such diet and diet groups can empower the harmful habit of overeating and increase your mental and emotional preoccupation with food. These diets have minimal use in the long term of weight management. You can lose weight on these diets initially, but they have to be life-long, which is not possible. It is also not empowering and they can be expensive.

Freedom of choice is lacking in the processed food of the Weight Watchers and the Slimfast Diet. The Slimfast diet manifests as a line of low-calorie drinks available in mainstream grocery stores. If you drink only them, you will lose weight, but you will not improve your overall health or your emotional state. You will not have permanence and you will not be truly empowered. While initially these planned meals may be useful for weight reduction, ultimately you will be better off dealing with your original causes of excess eating, develop your personal form of eating and eat for natural health.

*The **Detox Diets** claim to work by detoxing your body through colonics, ionic foot cleanses and skin cleansing. While detoxification is certainly important, it is only one element of total holistic health that I consider in order to find your healthy optimal weight. These diets also advocate more natural food and that is also an important step in the right direction. These diets often use juice and drinks as the only form of nutrients consumed during the diet. That can be harmful because anything in drink form usually means a large bolus of sugar in liquid state entering your body. Liquid-only consumption is not natural or helpful for diabetic concerns and mood stability, and is not something you can do permanently. While the protein part of the liquid drinks does tend to diminish the hunger response, often the quality of the protein drinks is suspect. And there is the missing element of dealing strategically with the original causes for people who become overweight.

*You—On a Diet is a very simple look at obesity from the traditional medical perspectives of calories, science of chemicals and fattening food. It talks a lot of the scientific findings of hormones and how they play in weight gain. Oddly enough, it is difficult to read with loads of sarcasm. Having a shotgun-like approach to presenting the latest scientific data on weight, it often seems to create a conflict in itself. Emotional issues are addressed superficially; issues that I believe must be dealt with individually and on a deeper level of psychology for permanence. The book places emotions in a category of being almost the results of body chemicals, giving a typical back seat modern medicine perspective to the reality and importance of the emotions and thoughts of the human mind. The stress levels make-up of the individual is mentioned, but they are not dealt with thoroughly or presented in this diet book in any way that would get any reader close to permanent weight loss. The authors specifically refer to the problem of self-esteem and the dieter. Well of course, but you can't stop by simply identifying a problem. You have to go much deeper and provide solutions and specific techniques for change which have eluded the authors of this book.

The same problem inherent in all trendy diets like this one

returns to haunt the dieter--and that is getting on a path of a truly altered lifestyle and a changed inner emotional and mental makeup.

The authors would like everyone to not make weight loss difficult and so encourage people not to look deeply into their lives. Not smart! The American public became overweight by not looking at what they were doing. When people *did* become aware of their excess weight, they looked at the least important factors --food, instead of looking at themselves.

Still, compared to other diet books published previously, this book attempts to cover a lot of information about weight that most diet books do not. The diet recommends canola oil which I consider a poison because it contains one percent euric acid, does not mention Hemoglobin A1c (which I consider a standard of diabetes monitoring); it recommends chocolate, coffee and alcohol, which I consider harmful damaging herbs or chemicals. They also embrace prescription drugs, bariatric surgery and almost all diet plans as if wanting to be accepted by all other diet businesses, which might be revealing to the framework and marketing of the book.

*There are hundreds of gimmicky diets with such deceptive advertising that their names are not worthy of mention. Some diet literature deceptively advertises that you'll lose your cellulite first, clearly an irresponsible attempt at this time to appeal to people who would like to believe this nonsense. Some diets claim that you will lose your tummy and hip fat first, which is never the case with any diet. A successful weight loss program takes time, but if it's a good program, that doesn't matter. Eventually, your heart and your life will have changed. The last pounds come off and with them, the cellulite and the last fat from the hips and tummy. On top of that, no diet will ever achieve optimal health and body proportion without significant exercise to sculpt the lean muscle mass optimal for function.

The Paleolithic Diet

The diet that I like the most if the diet alone were all that was needed is called the **Paleolithic Diet** and it involves a logical, evolutionary view of food. Based upon a re-creation of what mankind was eating 100,000 years ago, the diet has no cereal grains, no dairy and no refined sugars. All of these tend to be allergenic foods for some people today, so it is a very safe diet from that standpoint. While the diet may not go into enough detail for best individual food compatibility, it does get people thinking in the right direction. What you do eat in this diet are vegetables, fruits and nuts. In direct contrast to the Atkins Diet, it is pro vegetarian.

Most of these diets have come and gone and, in some cases, come again. The short term one pill, one diet approach to weight loss has proven itself to be impermanent, as shown by the constant release of new diets for our growing overweight majority. When you call your food intake a diet, you think of it as temporary.

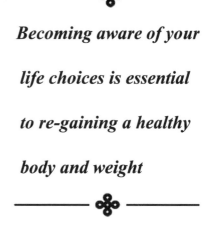

Becoming aware of your life choices is essential to re-gaining a healthy body and weight

I personally don't believe in dieting or calorie counting. I prefer to live more freely and "wholly." A diet is a prescribed eating program--something you have to do where health is not the end product. But a lifestyle change can permanently and happily affect your weight and life. Certainly you must educate yourself about food and nutrition in order to make informed decisions about your shopping, eating and food preparation. But it can be fun, all the new discoveries opening up a whole new menu in front of you.

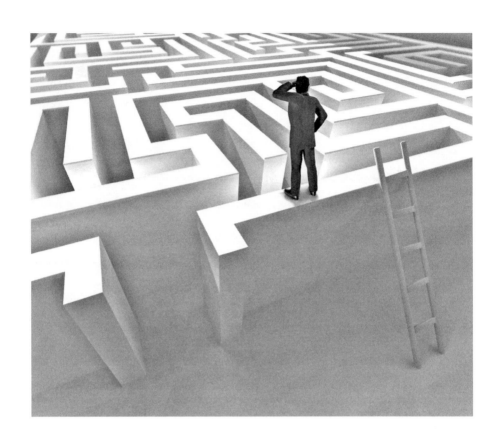

You know where you are now.

You know where you need to go.

Start

PART II:

Inside-Out Changes for Weight Loss

Chapter Three

Inside the Inside-Outside Diet

Warning! You are asking to take charge of *your* life, *your* choices, *your* behavior, and *your* health. This means everything you are, do and know! But you can't expect to be different without *being* different. Are you ready!

The *Inside-Out* part of this book starts the true "therapy of change," and may be the least familiar to many of you because it is the most missing element of basic human health in our educational system and culture. Therefore, I've given many examples of how emotional and mental changes occur for you to better grasp and implement the fundamentals of changing yourself.

The heart of the matter is that you eat the wrong foods at the wrong times for powerful inner emotional reasons. It isn't physical hunger—in fact, it isn't the body usually urging you to eat. Instead, it's your mind and emotions making demands to satisfy your emotional energy needs by eating, because of how you respond to the world around you. The heart of the matter is that freedom on the Outside comes from freedom on the Inside. Moderate self-discipline will equal self-mastery. Use this understanding of yourself with knowledge of food and nutrition to achieve the best health for your correct body size.

Why Inside-Outside? OK, let me ask you this: Why not pick up another weight-loss diet and follow it like the last 40 fad diets have suggested? Well, there you have it. Forty diets won't work long term because they weren't structured properly to deal with the highest priority as to what causes excess weight.

One physical mathematical equation we've told you reveals the mechanics of weight loss: the amount of calories you take in, divided by the amount of exercise calories you lose equals your weight gain or loss. But there is also a hidden *emotional equation* more powerful than the physical equation: the amount of pleasure in your life divided by the amount of stress in your life equals your final weight!

On still a deeper level, there is the hidden mental equation: your self-beliefs that empower you divided by your beliefs that counter you equals your final weight. The tendency to believe that you can express yourself freely, enjoy life and will survive--divided by the beliefs of self-doubt, low self-esteem and an unwillingness to change your habits equals your final body weight. If ever there was a case for the "weight" of emotions behind losing or gaining weight, this is it.

The answer? To really effect a deep and lasting improvement, the psychological and emotional you must be understood and altered. For example, you can change your job (and that may be very important), but the question would still go back to why you worked at such a stressful job—and will the new job turn out as stressful. Understanding and then changing yourself is the only approach to permanently correcting your overeating life cycle. You have to stop converting the stress energy of your life into eating energy, digestive energy and resulting body mass.

Reflect upon your day and determine how you feel when you reach for the food. Connect the role of stress or the need for pleasure to how that extra-large order of burger and fries affects your eating lifestyle. **Start noticing what you are *really* feeling right before you get that drive to eating.** *Are you bored? Are you stressed? Is it true hunger?*

Consider this: When you awake in the morning after 6 to 8 hours of sleeping--probably not having eaten for 12 hours--you awake without hunger. You might eat breakfast or share a family meal out of habit, or prepare for a laborious day with something to eat. But still, most people do not experience hunger when they awake in the morning. How could this be?

If you had a good night's sleep, your sleep cycle and dream state eliminated all your left-over emotional energies and unresolved thoughts from the day before. As you awake with an empty mind and peaceful emotional state, you also do not feel the need to eat. But for most of us, this overnight cleansing does not last. Instead, it just takes a few hours or minutes of anxiety or worry about anticipated obligations and you're ready to be distracted from the thought of tackling those activities by eating. Usually this starts at work.

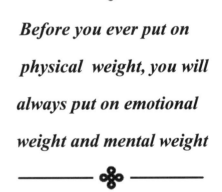

Before you ever put on physical weight, you will always put on emotional weight and mental weight

As the day of stresses goes along further, with added decisions and emotional interplay that keep us on our toes, we believe ourselves to be "hungry." Next step: We eat according to our culture or our ingrained habits. We look for an escape or distraction from conflict, even if that conflict is totally within us. We have more decisions pending, more stresses perceived and further ill emotions flowing. We want to devour something, take a break with a cup of coffee, eat something chewy and sweet; and experience the uplifting or distracting activity of eating. Eating is the emotionally safest and easiest, socially acceptable programmed habit. We might think we are hungry but often we are not, or at least not to the degree to which we then eat. Shake, stir and repeat every day for years and you have excess weight and an unhealthy, diminished life.

Eating when you're *not* hungry is a learned response to calm stress and alleviate boredom. By the end of a waking day, unresolved drives turn into distracting drives to eat so you can calm and appease yourself. What you didn't deal with during the day--such as, conflicts, concerns, doubts, what you need to accomplish and have not--remains an overriding feeling that makes you yearn for pleasure and peace, as found in food. The connection between your thoughts, emotions, drives and overeating is very direct. **Thoughts and emotions are, and always will be, the original cause of overeating.**

The truth is we're hard-wired to feel satisfied by eating. Being human, it is a reflexive evolutionary trait important for the need to survive. We have hormonal feedback that tells us to eat, and sugar is probably the biggest chemical that generates pleasure within us, but it is temporary and certainly damaging in excess, i.e. diabetes.

Before you ever put on any physical excess weight, you will always put on emotional weight and mental weight. Call it stress or burdens, boredom or dis-ease--either way you examine the phenomenon, it is damaging. When life makes you overweight, you need to look at how you live your life. You need to learn why you're going round and round, day after day, with the same damaging habits accumulating emotional debt.

When I talk about losing the emotional weight, most women consider this the predominant feelings that hold them back. Men may identify themselves more with what they think and do. Both attitudes are true aspects of who you are and both attitudes need to be examined when change and weight loss are your goals.

A **mental goal** for you might be to remove a specific negative self-concept about yourself by acknowledging when it started, where it came from and doing self-talk to affirm a new self opinion. An **emotional goal** might be to feel and emit positivism throughout your day as you interact in the world. How many days can you go without commenting with a negative emotion and thought?

Are you dissatisfied? Is your pleasure meter running chronically low? Have you had to install a second tension meter due to the stress you find yourself involved with in life? Has another internal drive gotten you so involved in business and financial affairs that you are living a discontented life? Why aren't you succeeding or happy? Why can't you find the time to enjoy exercise? What part of you is interfering with your more simple peaceful nature?

Most people are doing unfulfilling things in their lives which is a source of stress and chronic boredom

It's easy to be distracted by the often confusing surroundings of a busy life so that you never notice yourself playing the overeating food games of pleasure and distraction. No one can stop you but you. Keep that in mind. You have to slow down. Rarely do life events force us to become completely aware of our destructive inner behaviors. You can set certain stop points in your life to re-evaluate your choices, thoughts, beliefs, emotions, pursuits and directions in life. Simply becoming aware of the emotional triggers that make you overeat will give you opportunity to re-direct your choices away from eating as a means of expending emotional energy.

When you are sad, stressed or even bored, you typically start to look ahead to something pleasurable. So you usually think about eating something, away from threats or stress, away from people. You think home, alone and a TV that consoles us. You don't think about sharing your problems or becoming more sociable. Anything that distracts you from the unpleasantness churning in your mind feels preferable as a way out, rather than facing the issues.

Eating is a common distraction. This is a natural drive for many people--sidestepping difficulties and hoping that avoidance will make you feel better. For the moment, inwardly, it feels right. Outwardly, though, it can lead to overeating as a compensating mechanism. Often these stressful situations are something we should have never gotten into in the first place. However, what led us to these stresses is that we thought we needed to take on some event to survive or live. When you start to tear down the emotional mechanisms responsible for gaining weight, you will be able to see how seemingly trivial moments of rewards, games and pleasures play out in your daily life.

The good news is that there are techniques to find and change the damaging internal beliefs, discordant emotions and errant drives that keep sabotaging you. First of all, know that damaging internal beliefs are those that create emotions of stress or do not allow peace of mind to flow from you. The *Inside-Outside* emotional healing techniques will help you change this. They will fulfill and balance pleasure, dispel tension energy, and help you remember what a peaceful feeling is. You'll find out why you manufacture tension and what it does to your urge to eat.

The *Inside-Outside* Plan to lose the mental weight, lose the emotional weight and lose the physical weight begins with you. Because people are best able to take in only a few steps at a time, it is best to have only one or two key emotional, mental, physical and lifestyle goals to achieve each week. Once you obtain some knowledge and incorporate changes into your life, you can go on to add other pieces of awareness and make further improvements to yourself.

The *Outside-Inside* food, supplements, herbs and exercise tricks to weight loss found in Part 3 of this book are the easiest to put in motion because they require the least understanding and willpower to do. Start by making these physical changes in your lifestyle and you'll immediately improve your mood, clarity and willpower. With this beginning strength you can start to adjust your emotional and mental origins of overeating. Correct the outer and inner causes of excess weight and you'll improve daily. With this blueprint for success you need to know:

*It is a long commitment to healthy weight, not a 10-day antibiotic treatment where you're cured and done. You have to be patient. It will take *one year for you to change your Outside and Inside health* so that new thinking is ingrained within you and to make lasting changes in your body and psyche. This course of your life will not be a straight line of success but a zigzag back and forth improvement that will probably include surfacing episodes of old habits of poor eating and damaging food memories. It is the overall direction that must be accepted in your pursuit of health and optimal weight.

*It will require effort on your behalf, to know yourself and explore what is going on within your body, mind and lifestyle. You will have to do some things differently than you have ever done before.

*It will require you to change yourself in a good way. So be prepared to be different.

*Your lifestyle will inevitably have to be different in terms of how you live your life and spend your day. Expect your 24 hour clock and weekly calendar to be reset–they must, so start now.

*You will need to monitor your health for safety. This means potential doctor visits or simply purchasing and using chemstrips if you decide to use fasting during your evolution of body and mind.

***Your relationships will change**. Your relationship of you to yourself, you to family, you to work, you to food, you to your perspective to live life, you to spirit and nature, you to stress and you to happiness.

*We all get distracted by family and work, and our very memory will often kick in responses to old ways of acting and dealing with emotions by eating when we are caught with our energy out of our comfort zone. Setting physical, emotional and mental goals along with a lifestyle maintenance program to keep you on track will simplify your schedule and minimize your distractions.

*There is room to individualize your path to a healthy body.

*Although I never initially recommend weight-loss products as a way to permanent weight loss, in some cases, if you've already started a program with meal replacements from various manufacturers, you can continue them a few weeks to give you time to educate yourself about natural foods. Try these replacement drinks and foods for a few weeks and then come off any of these plans when you are ready to establish your individual, natural whole food eating.

Or, you can simply start to add better foods and remove damaging foods from your "best foods list" for your health, eventually implementing your food choices from a natural low-fat, low-carb, predominantly vegetarian, Paleolithic wholesome food program. It is *not* knowing what you can eat, what to buy and how to prepare better foods that allows people to slip back into old harmful food consumption.

Plan ahead and don't put yourself down even if you do occasionally go back to old ways or foods before you can pull yourself out of it. Getting down on yourself will not help you as negativity usually deteriorates your best energy level. Unhealthy energy levels cause drives to eat and are part of the cycle of thoughts that develop distressed emotions that lead to bad food.

Food, like many things we experience in life, have meanings to us that are more than the substance itself. Food can equal security, joy and peace.

Ultimately, you have to want to be more happy than you want to be sad. You have to be in cooperation with life and people more than in conflict. You need to be more in peace than turmoil. It does start with you.

The Vitality of Youth

can be regained

when you put

your true emotional

core

back into your life

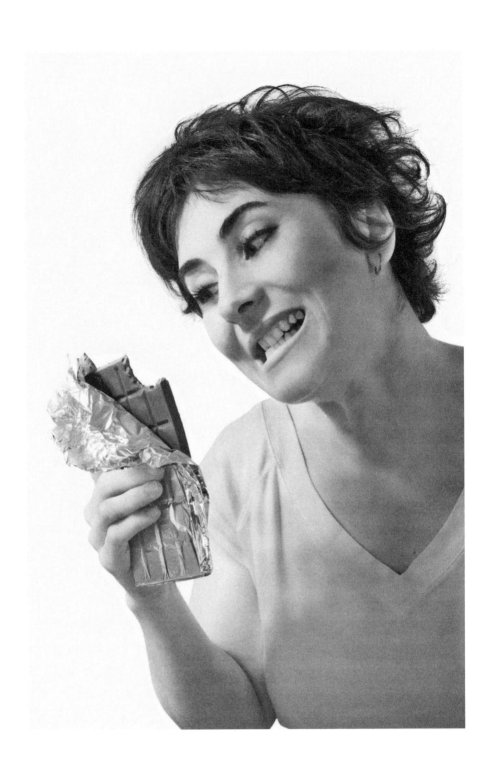

Chapter Four

Losing the Emotional Weight

<u>Breaking the Code to Your Emotions</u>

We all have emotions. You cannot be alive in this world without them. Emotions generate spontaneously whenever we interact with anything in the environment. People, places and things all generate feelings and emotions within us when we respond to them, touch, feel, hear sounds and feel vibrations. Emotions generate as a means of communicating. Emotions are forms of energy that travel around your body and through it, reaching out to anyone or anything around you. Your emotions have different quantities and qualities. Everyone has the same types of emotions, generated the same way, given off and felt by others, but revealed and sensed in a very personal manner. **An essential part of the *Inside-Outside* diet is for you to determine what emotions you are in need of, or are generating as they relate to overeating.**

<u>Overeating Due to Stress</u>

Where does appetite come from and does it have anything to do with emotions? Appetite is both a feeling and a drive to consume food and alter energy. But, stress can both suppress and increase appetite depending upon how you learn to manage it. Connect emotion and food and you'll find that **people primarily overeat as a means to relieve, dump or balance emotional stress and anxiety**.

This is the main pattern we can point to for why people overeat and become overweight in the United States. Let's look at this powerful overeating mechanism more closely to understand it. Increased stress at home or work, usually because of frustration, worry, disappointment or a clash of personalities in your environment, results in eating for relief or as a means of reward from excessive negativity. Our progressive, fast-paced culture provides continual pressures on us to perform that result in excess stress. When that happens *we don't feel well* and we look for ways to return our elevated anxious energy to a comfortable feeling. We often don't know this is what we're doing.

Stress is a multi-dimensional reaction that can arise because of fear. It also arises from your belief that some conflict at work or at home has greater importance and value than maintaining peace and joy. When your will is challenged by personal conflicts or life circumstances, you have a physical reaction. You feel your energy go up as the release of adrenal hormones, cortisol and glutamate all prepare your body for action. With this higher energy level, as caused by conflicting emotions, you feel uncomfortable--even insecure--and that biological survival kicks in.

At these moments, some people increase their agitation to fight. Others give up, become depressed and feel hopeless, thereby dropping their overall energy levels without truly correcting their original troubling beliefs. Either response to distress doesn't feel peaceful. We consciously reach for the foods that will raise or lower our energy to make us feel normal and reassured again. **People are constantly altering their energy to feel better.**

Many mood altering foods cause "bottoming out" stress situations where your energy first goes high then drops very low and these foods are to be avoided! Sugar is the biggest culprit, creating a feeling of security and comfort. Monosodium glutamate (msg) and individual food allergens are other products that disrupt our normal energy. Fats drain a lot of the liver's energy in digesting a fatty meal - and many people love butter and deep-fried foods for how it settles their excess energy down.

Eating chewy meat releases tension in the jaw. Other foods that release tension energy are chocolate, which tends to lower your energy level and can even act as a depressant. Alcohol first releases tension and then lowers energy. These are the subtle inward effects that overeaters have constantly in play when they deal with stress events in their life.

Stress is a state we often connect with our jobs, which we tie into survival. Many people are working the wrong job, and doing the wrong thing in life. That is an ultimate cause of disease.

Then again, stress arises from how you negotiate the world, reveal your personality, your strengths and weaknesses on the job or at home--in which case, make those changes to yourself and not look to others to keep the pressure off you. Find a way to make your life work so it's not perceived as stressful and thus generate the damaging neuro-hormonal cortisol responses which can compel you to relieve this energy by overindulgent repetitive eating.

People in high-stress occupations, or those who struggle to emotionally manage their affairs, all generate cortisol, dopamine, glutamate and adrenaline in their blood and neurohormonal systems. These fight or flight impulses want to be released and satisfied. If you're not emotionally balanced, discharged or fulfilled, that dissatisfaction is misappropriated from a natural release to that of eating. It's the default setting of consumptive overeating for those who eat to settle down after stress has built up by the end of their day.

Overeating isn't the only way people handle negative stress. For example, you can go into depression, drink alcohol excessively or drive recklessly. Other problems frequently exist with overeating and you need to holistically address all the ramifications that spill off a stressed lifestyle and mind.

While discharging an emotion is one key to health, sometimes it is difficult to discharge an emotion on the job without consequences.

The Inside Outside Diet

Fortunately, imagination, mind games and time away from work that can help you do this are unseen and unheard. No one will know when you are redirecting stress or fulfilling pleasure from within. You can release that emotional excess after work by kicking a ball around and letting the irritation out, or do some of the emotional exercises that bring relief to your emotional nature. Discharging emotions by biting, chewing and gulping foods is not helpful. This sets lifestyle patterns and habits for future repetition that are part of the mechanism for gaining weight in the first place. They have already been part of your emotional cycle of weight gain and disease. *Identifying* your specific emotional energies that lead to overeating is one important step to fixing your problem.

Transmute stress energy into eating and digestion and you feel better for the moment, but do this every day, and yes, you put on weight. You can only do this a few times before the energy of stress is transmuted into pounds of excess body mass, a conversion of E=mc squared. This emotional tension can actually be stored in your body and be awaiting release for years. Disturbing emotional stresses unreleased and stored within parts of your physical body can account for restless sleep and bodily dysfunction even years later in life.

Your body is made to respond to your emotions. Emotions are only bad when they are too constant, too extreme or not released. When your immediate reaction to emotions you cannot cope with become fast food to the stomach you pay the price later. Fast food satisfies briefly but makes you ill and overweight in the long run. Eventually, physical sickness ensues.

When you have a lot of stress in your Outside life, such as at work, you tend to come home and wall off your feelings even from yourself with video games or television. Stop here and make this change in your lifestyle:

First, counter the Outside stressors by making yourself be outgoing and not indulging in the indwelling activities which continue to close you off. Find other routes for emotional discharge such as physical activity like exercise or emotional exercises that make you feel more balanced. Instead of numbing your sensations, engage yourself privately, directly or even socially to experience healthy body awareness.

Second, you must consider if the interactions you are involved in are the right ones for you. Try to make stress-lessening changes to the job itself or how you *perceive* the job when working. If it is not the right vocation, make your best plan and preparations and leave it for what you really want to do. That could be another job, and independent job, school, or the same work with a new employer. If the real culprits are your own responses to how your work affects you, then you must look into your very mind to change that–*and it can be done.*

People Overeat Because of a Need for Pleasure

All human beings have basic emotional core drives for companionship, stimulation, creativity, security and pleasure. Cookies and milk have always been used to nurture security and pleasure. If you are psychologically deprived of pleasure, bored or too emotionally protected, you may become an overeater and over-consume food as a substitute for providing the pleasure you both lack, and need.

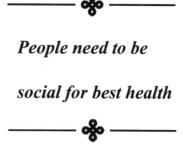

People need to be

social for best health

Eating is a safe pleasure-- it doesn't bite you back for some time until you become very overweight.

Risking little exposure, you can eat in the personal confines and safety of your car (drive-throughs) or at home, without anyone yelling at you, telling you what to do or in anyway inserting any negativity into that bite of food. You can eat in a controlled environment which in itself is a drive for security. Eating stops all the talking and the very form of communication that may be your usual source of agitation. If this describes you, excess eating is about pleasure and security. Overeating from a deprived emotional lifestyle can exist with stress eating or by itself. Which are you?

Emotional Starvation

People are starved for non-edible pleasure in their lives. Non-edible pleasure refers to activities, hobbies and social interactions where food is neither sustenance nor empty calories. What gives you pleasure depends on how you look at life itself, and the degree to which you are capable of *feeling* pleasure. If you don't allow yourself to feel pleasure, or if you don't initiate actions that bring you pleasure, then you will be starved for it. This is because "feeling" something and having joy are natural core drives – everyone has them. Yet everyone will, at some point, begin to consume their pleasure through food when they fall below their satisfaction level of pleasure or joy. Their need for this energy demands it from their very core.

Even if you manage to rid yourself of financial stress, often you can end up after work, after kids, after family, never having the life or joy in life that your nature demands. The truth is that life often has moments and episodes where life is simply basic and boring. If you can't control your mind's actions or initiate peace within, you'll crawl around the world in search of pleasure. If you don't find it or don't allow it, you'll eat it.

You also need to relax emotionally, *not take everything as a crisis or disaster and keep setbacks and disappointments in perspective.* Stop brooding over what you cannot change. Keep in mind the spiritual truth that often "negative" things happen to move us along to what we would probably otherwise not do or learn. Reminding yourself of this is important because it can keep you in a positive, optimistic energy state, even when "bad" things happen. Pessimistic thinking generates discordant emotions of stress or depression which can manifest in overeating as a recovering means to feeling good again.

Allow yourself to feel pleasure and let yourself feel vulnerable with others to feel more pleasure. If you feel emotionally starved, exposing yourself to the small pleasures of being with friends, helping others, tossing a ball with your son are all real life pleasures. Consciously remind yourself to engage with people and things. Interacting with people in non-threatening play modes naturally returns most people to a nice comfort zone. On a bigger scale, reinvent your dreams; reset your daily lifestyle and how you emotionally interplay in your interactions in life.

Of course, you didn't just get to this point without a history. Strong imprints from your childhood about giving and receiving pleasure can perpetuate the feeling now of being emotionally starved. For example, maybe you grew up with parents who were unaffectionate and controlled your feelings of pleasure by making you feel guilty or "bad." It is mislearned behavior that has morphed into the form of altered emotions and choices you live with now. Take control of it! You can re-program your mind.

Instead of feeling pleasure with others or through events, eating became the substitute. Eating out of a need to feel secure in your pleasure can navigate your life into a shipwreck. In this case you will have to intentionally navigate your way back to an emotionally rewarding life.

What does this all have to do with being overweight? Everything, for many people! Blocked emotions, unexpressed emotions and limitations of emotional expression (not that it isn't sometimes necessary) will cause tension in your body that will find release if not in overeating, then through other deviations of behavior. You can spend your emotions digesting food or you can digest what you have learned and release unwanted emotions through non-edible means like exercise, socializing, meditation or intentional healing exercises.

If you think that ignoring the people and world around you can protect you from developing deviate eating and self-harmful behavior, you are wrong. Many secluded or sensitive people have become reclusive only to find that their universal core drives of creativity, sharing, and pleasure lead them to eat everything around them. Their physical health and body deteriorates along with their isolationist thinking. People need to be social for best health. Being with others in an open, innocent and intimate way--intimate in terms of emotional connection with others-- are core drives to being alive.

Every behavior you act on started out by serving a purpose. For example, there are behaviors that ensure survival, surety, pain avoidance, fear avoidance, and energy stabilization which is vulnerability protection. Behaviors have correlating emotions.

Getting rid of the negative emotions still harbored in your body from anything in your past is important for your health. The only thing worse than constantly generating negative emotions from the way you think is by *not* releasing the ones retained in your body and mind from the past (Yes, it is common.)

Tension and specific energy related to personal conflicts can be stored in your cells from your past. It is as if part of your mind never realized the danger has passed and it continues to manifest "alarm" as if a threat was current. If unresolved conflicts build it up and are never released, it causes outright physical illness over time.

When you contemplate your lifestyle, it will reveal what types of emotions you are experiencing and the choices you are making, specifically, in terms of your relationship to food. This gives you the opportunity to explore how you function and allows you the opportunity to start making significant changes to your choices. This will improve the impact of your emotional imprints on your weight and health. *Identification* of your choices and sensitivities is the beginning process of accomplishing this. To start making changes, you'll need to pay close attention to when and how you eat. Try this:

*For one week, start taking a daily inventory where you write down when you eat and what you were feeling <u>before</u> you ate. Did you feel needy, stressed, frustrated, bored, depressed, or did you eat out of habit?

*Then, write down how you felt <u>after</u> eating, what you ate and how much. This will help you to understand your emotional links to overeating. This might seem like a slow process, but if you are overweight, you have been making unconscious decisions to eat emotionally. You can be aware of these links without writing them down once you identify thoroughly what you are doing, but I find a reviewable record of your emotional eating has more impact than just recall. The written record speaks for itself.

And remember: if you're overweight, your mind is already not paying attention, and you can "forget" or deny what you consumed in a day. Committing to this plan will help you as "your" plan has already not worked for you in the life that got you overweight. Afterwards, you'll be fully in charge of yourself more than you ever realized.

*Go deeper and be specific with the information you're writing down about your food intake. Determine if you overeat out of a need for pleasure or a need to dump stress or both. Determine when in the day you are most likely to use food to correct your energy and you'll be prepared to counter the old urges with new techniques, such as walking or by substituting out high-sugar snacks with healthier ones that, in some cases, you can prepare ahead of time.

Keeping a journal can help you link your emotional and mental reasons for overeating with the foods you physically eat as a response. Let me tell you more by sharing with you this story: A patient who'd gained 60 pounds told me that she didn't know where some of the weight came from since she didn't really overeat every day. By keeping a journal, she was stunned to discover that she was an "unconscious" eater. She'd clean her kids' plates, dip into the chips with her husband when he watched TV, have a Snickers bar when she carpooled--and "forgot about what she'd eaten after it was gone." She saw how she'd been fooling herself by unconsciously consuming and discounting snacks and scraps from her kids' plates as being "real food." The journal also helped her see why she was snacking and denying it--stress at home that she had been denying. After identifying the times, means and origins of her overeating, she was able to begin to counter and resolve her original issues more clearly.

When you're not comfortable expressing blocked emotions you can learn to let them out gradually. Understand exactly which feelings are building up inside you. Strongly-held beliefs that block your emotions and your ability to grow emotionally may need a professional therapist to guide you through both empathetically and efficiently. That in-depth therapeutic approach helps you understand how you came to behave or feel a certain way while still keeping your cognition current. Helpful therapy from a professional, who might see yourself more clearly than your own mind, may provide a way to free you up from your own mental confusion. Don't be afraid to seek professional help if you become stalled.

Understanding your nature is helped and helped powerfully when you are alone and focused on contemplating your life. In the end, of course, you must become a person of the world. You can not make your own version of a successful Neverland. The healthy outcome is to eventually be an open Everland, where you are complete, totally aware and capable of dealing with emotional challenges and personal sensitivities that often get bruised. When you gain a truer and healthier perspective of your worth, and who you are, you'll stabilize both your emotions and your necessary emotional vulnerability in the world.

Actively implement positive emotions *consciously* by doing life-affirming activities, such as taking a walk in the park, and consciously enjoying it. Feel it fully aware. Allow the wind, the leaves and the vibrant animals to enter your positive consciousness. Know what is really important in your life. You will need to remind yourself of the inner happiness you need and willfully allow yourself to *feel* happiness if this has been your key block to health. **Use the emotionally healing exercises to help you remember what joyful living emotions are like.**

Negative stress comes from the root cause of fear for your survival. What's most important is that you change the survival thought that drives you to the bad food, and understand what makes you develop so much tension energy. Dump tension energy through non-eating means, especially if eating has been your pattern of coping with tension. You could use a punching pillow, establish a walking route near where you live, buy a gym membership or find a partner who's going through what you are for added support. Do anything but turn to food to dissipate your tension energy. **This is where you need to implement a strategic back-up means for releasing excess negative energy day or night.** Having a stuctured plan prevents unnecessary eating.

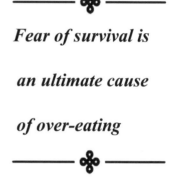

Fear of survival is an ultimate cause of over-eating

Individualize your plan, but it must be effective in dumping food-focused energy once you build it up. In fact, the fastest weight loss you'll experience without fasting is to consciously make a plan and convert every calorie-gaining emotional eating moment to a calorie burning physical exercise for release. Instead of gaining pounds at that moment of temptation, you can transmute that energy into calories lost--a win-win situation. Figure out your activity plan ahead of time or you could be caught off guard. Your short term memory, which rules such behaviors, such as eating to release stress, will take precedence and be re-enacted if you don't make a plan ahead of time to deal with it. Once the compulsion energy of binge eating becomes high, it will often be too difficult to stop and "think" of a different way of dumping it–unless you've made a plan beforehand.

A problem for many people with tension energy isn't the negativity, but that the energy is uncomfortably too high. People get used to their energy levels in a comfort zone as it is associated with vulnerability when too high and depression when too low. Eating is a way for you to use that excess energy by digesting food and consequently lowering your energy. You feel better after eating a very large meal either with a high fat content or a high-glycemic load.

For many people, overeating is in reality an energy-adjusting response they unconsciously initiate as a response to relieve uncomfortable energy. Look at the diagram of energy, moods, food and remedies on the following page as often a picture is worth a thousand words.

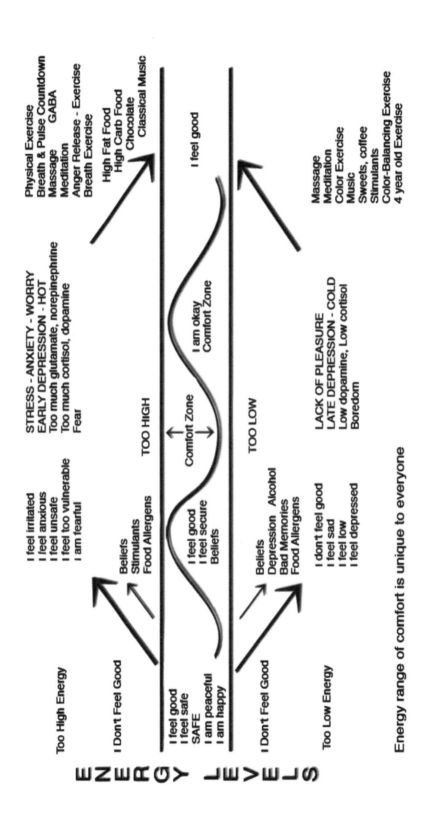

ENERGY LEVELS

Too High Energy

I Don't Feel Good

I feel irritated
I feel anxious
I feel unsafe
I feel too vulnerable
I am fearful

Beliefs
Stimulants
Food Allergens

STRESS - ANXIETY - WORRY
EARLY DEPRESSION - HOT
Too much glutamate, norepinephrine
Too much cortisol, dopamine
Fear

TOO HIGH

Physical Exercise
Breath & Pulse Countdown
Massage   GABA
Meditation
Anger Release - Exercise
Breath Exercise

High Fat Food
High Carb Food
Chocolate
Classical Music

Comfort Zone ↔ Comfort Zone

I am okay
Comfort Zone

I feel good
I feel secure
Beliefs

I feel good

I feel good
I feel safe
SAFE
I am peaceful
I am happy

Beliefs
Depression Alcohol
Bad Memories
Food Allergens

I don't feel good
I feel sad
I feel low
I feel depressed

LACK OF PLEASURE
LATE DEPRESSION - COLD
Low dopamine, Low cortisol
Boredom

TOO LOW

Too Low Energy

I Don't Feel Good

Massage
Meditation
Color Exercise
Music
Sweets, coffee
Stimulants
Color-Balancing Exercise
4 year old Exercise

Energy range of comfort is unique to everyone

The Inside Outside Diet

We all live within energy levels, high to low, where we feel most comfortable. But energy can be higher or much lower than where we feel peaceful and secure. Within our comfort energy range we experience ups and downs and can still feel basically okay. If our energy exceeds our top level we don't feel right. The same thing happens when our energy

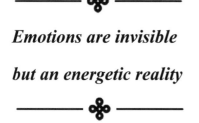

Emotions are invisible

but an energetic reality

goes too low, we don't feel right, either. When our energy levels go beyond our comfort range, we may subconsciously try to move our energy back to "normal" and feel better. Our memories contain the imprints of how we have learned to do this from our past. If you are overweight, food has been a tool you have used to adjust your energy.

There are outside factors that move our energy up and down and inside factors that do the same. Certain stimulants and foods can move our energy higher. Caffeine, high dose sugar, msg, certain amino acids all move our energy up. High fat foods, high carbohydrate foods, chocolate and alcohol can take our energy downward. Personal food allergens or incompatible foods can take our energy up or down. Outside stimulating events and people can take our energy uncomfortably too high where outside people and events can bring anger and fear to us as a form of stress. Most importantly, your very beliefs and thoughts form the springboard for generating energy as you respond to any event in your life.

Similar factors can drop your energy levels and again we don't feel right. Knowledge of certain foods, supplements effects and knowing how you respond can all keep you from exceeding your energy comfort zone or at least return you to normal quickly. Once you go out of your comfort zone, knowledge of certain techniques like the emotional healing exercises, massage, classical music, meditation, supplements, better foods, and physical exercises can return you to your comfort zone.

By far, most of the ways you've subconsciously returned yourself to a normal comfort range energy has been by food. Certain foods absorb your excess stress energy and drop your energy back to normal. Other foods stimulate you when your energy is low and pick you up to a comfortable emotional energy. The problem with food besides extra weight eventually is that they wear off and our mental, emotional and lifestyle ways repeat again and again--all going from "I don't feel right," to "I feel okay" again. Recognizing your patterns using this energy diagram may help you take control of what you are doing with food and create other means to bring "comfort" to your life. **Learn how to alter your energy without eating.**

One solution, in part, is that you can learn to alter your energy to be higher than you are used to feeling. This must be done in a relaxed way. By simply realizing that what you are feeling is higher energy due to tension, and not a life-threatening situation you are a step ahead.

Try this energy exercise to convert stress to comfort:

<u>The Ascending energy visualization</u>

Breathe deeply, relax and consciously feel your excess energy in your body. You can often sense it as tightness in your chest. You can close your eyes if it helps your ability to feel. Let your energy rise naturally through your chest and up your neck and into your head like mercury ascending in a thermometer. Consciously *relax* as you feel the higher energy in your body. Don't fight the feeling but let it travel. As you allow that energy to rise and expand, you will feel less tense. Visualize and feel tingling in your body where the energy resides and where it wants to go. Let the energy rise out of the top of your head if it wants to go higher but stay connected with it.

Often, when you relax and let the energy find its place, you'll discover that the uncomfortable drive to eat or dump energy will dissipate. This is "transmuting energy," or energy you can change. The key to this technique is relaxing, not fighting the tension and allowing the feeling to expand and rise.

Emotions are invisible but real. They are true packets of willful energy that have a reality that must be expressed and used. Don't discount your emotional feelings; understand them, see where they come from and find new ways to use them. If your emotions are too destructive, too harmful, or too negative, then you'll have to dig deep until you figure out why you generate them. This kind of self knowledge can only help you know your thoughts and beliefs much better. Your thoughts and beliefs will always reveal how you respond to your living environment and why you generate the emotions that you do.

Living the right lifestyle with the positive attitudes generates the more positive emotions. That lifestyle develops from what you consciously and unconsciously think. For example, many cancer patients are known to have gone through a very distressing or depressing situation in the few years preceding their having cancer. Extreme stress and distress can, for some, generate overt physical disease.

Inner work and emotional exercises are done to put you in contact with your feelings and emotions--which you are constantly producing. The technique used to internally search the beliefs that set you in motion is *contemplation*, talked about in later chapters, and also in my book *Start Living...* You need to see what habits you have and why you continue to repeat them. Knowing how much you generate, in terms of negative emotions that urge you to eat, will tell you that undermining tension is not necessary so end it!

Vulnerability is an invisible dynamic of your consciousness that controls sensual emotional energy as it flows from and to you.

People tend to be sensually deprived by their own limitations. Natural emotional drives must interact through this personal vulnerability portal. Vulnerability can be either consciously or subconsciously controlled. Emotional-awareness exercises help open your capability to move energy, but you can tap into this ability by simply being aware of its existence and allowing emotional interaction when you feel yourself closing down. This can save you from developing an emotional burden.

If you have a fear of being hurt and have closed off your vulnerability, you can't experience pleasure from normal interactions and activities that could be rewarding. The ability to experience pleasure depends on your beliefs and perception of your experiences, coupled with your emotional vulnerability.

Your Drives

All human beings have some core human drives, and most people have a drive to feel pleasure instead of pain. You live your life to accomplish your drives, and, they can be manipulated, avoided or altered. This can happen willfully and consciously or unwillfully and subconsciously. I'm concerned here with the willful and conscious method of altering your drives so that they are self-fulfilling, selfless and pleasurable.

Fear of vulnerability can be a tension energy builder. Increased fear also increases the kind of emotional agitation that keeps you from moving into positive thinking or consciousness. Fear is responsible for many problems not being resolved. It is an internalized view of your survival as being threatened and in your believing in a negative outcome. It takes a lot of courage to keep the emotion of fear steady and in control so that fear transcends to faith.

We are individuals who each live different lives and yet we all create other drives that affect our cycles of thinking, emotions and worldly interactions. The basic human drives in regards to eating are a need to have pleasure or joy as we have mentioned, but also a need to be creative and express ourselves, a need to be socially interactive--to receive energy from others. We also have a need to be peaceful, a need to be entertained, a need to feel secure and a need to avoid feelings of fear. All these basic common drives occur along with your personal drives you've taken on due to your unique upbringing.

Any of these drives can be diverted into the eating and overweight cycle of living. You can see how evident this is when you think about appetite and appetite control. Appetite is about the urge to alter energy and satisfy hunger. You may say that you're overweight because you have a naturally big appetite. Appetite control focuses on altering your perception of being hungry and what you need to satisfy hunger

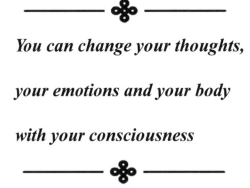

You can change your thoughts, your emotions and your body with your consciousness

urges, while allaying the desire to decrease stress.

Sometimes, the anxiety to finish unpleasant work as fast as possible is accompanied by constant snacking or carries over into rush meals. You eat quickly, distracted, with a lack of patience for a really good meal. You may go for fast food, an almost universally poor choice. Work on your attention span and develop more patience to improve this situation.

Western culture is largely devoid of the concept that you can alter, control and manipulate your emotions, thoughts and drives to create a "self" as you choose. Sure, implanted reflexes of living and eating instilled in you when you were more emotionally receptive may take precedence for a while, but you can remake them all with attention, persistence and time. While neuro-hormonal interactions are occurring inside your body that correlate to emotions and beliefs, *you* are not your hormones. You are affected by your hormones, you can affect your hormones--you are more than your hormones.

Begin considering these questions:

*What are the pleasures of your life?

*Do you remember feeling intimacy, happiness or peacefulness? What or to whom are these memories connected?

*Has constant agitation replaced your natural drives for feeling happy?

*What goals in life are you really pursuing?

*How much fun do you really experience with others, or is it a shell of a game that you live to get ahead? Can you socialize with people without eating for interaction?

*Can you consider your drives as they have shaped your life and decide how you want your drives to shape your future.

If you just ate when you felt true hunger, you wouldn't be overweight. If you weren't stressed so highly at home or work, you wouldn't compensate by eating huge meals or mood-altering beverages. If you're content with your energy and state of life you wouldn't be compelled to snack at all. Your own beliefs and self-opinions will consequently generate the anxiety or limit your interaction in the world. If you had a creative expressive life and could be doing more of what makes you happy, you'd see the immediate change: you wouldn't gorge for pleasure or snack so you have something to do, or be overweight.

Relationships:

You have relationships that are, for example, you to yourself, you to spouse or partner, you to family, you to work, you to friends, you to your environment, and you to spirituality. Another aspect of your emotional life is your relationship to adversity and the manufacture of emotions. Within each of these dynamics is the potential for peace or conflict. Any of these relationships can have negative beliefs that generate negative emotions that disrupt your health and lead to excess weight as a spill-over. When you think, "you can't handle it," or that "you're overwhelmed," or that "you're in jeopardy," you will generate stress energy. If a relationship becomes more about a lack of pleasure in your life with an increased amount of stress, you need to change the relationship or how you participate in that relationship. You see the relationship and, although a tougher task, see what you might be contributing to that stress.

When a relationship makes you uncomfortable, you feel the stress in your hands, your jaw and neck as they become tight. Be aware of these locations for holding tension. While you're figuring out how to improve or change a problematic relationship, you don't have to give in to the negativity. Instead, do physical relaxation and de-stressing exercises to release the self-sabotaging energy. These exercises help prevent you from eating for relief.

Emotional Exercises to Balance Energy and Relieve Stress

The following exercises will help you to return to an emotionally balanced state. As a result, you will be physically healthier.

Tension-Releasing Exercise

Starting with your hands, bend and stretch your fingers and wrists using a full range of motion to each part. After bending your fingers and wrist in full extension and flexion, lightly shake your hands to relax them.

Next, deal with your jaw by taking your index finger and thumb and slightly stretch your jaw open. Release and massage the masseter muscles on the sides of your jaw with your fingers and move your jaw back and forth in an easy manner to relax it.

Now deal with your neck. Start by massaging the back of your neck with your hands for at least a minute. Then slowly roll your head around to the left twice, and back to the right twice. Bend your head to the left and then to the right. Next, turn your head to the left and then to the right. Always go very slowly with neck exercises, and avoid all quick jerky movements. This will release the tension from your neck.

Massage the area from your neck to your shoulders where tension energy travels for action. Gently move your shoulders back, up and forward in a circle and them back the other way again.

Remember: All the emotional balancing exercises in this book are used to restore *natural* expressive emotions and body conditions.

The following is a good exercise for relaxing and de-stressing your body, which is one of many exercises from my book, *Start Living Stop Dying, 10 Steps to Natural Health.*

The Breath and Pulse Countdown Exercise

This exercise, like the previous one, will reduce your level of stress. In addition, it will help your body develop the ability to respond more easily to your thoughts and feelings. You will increase your body-awareness while putting yourself into a deep, restful state, which will also prepare you for whatever kind of follow-up technique, such as biofeedback, you may ever need to do. This exercise takes 10 to 20 minutes.

Assume a comfortable position. Begin to focus on your breathing, preferably breathing through your nose. Begin to concentrate less directly on your breathing but sense your chest moving up and down. The natural way to breathe is from very deep in the abdomen, so as you relax, your breathing will shift from your chest to deeper abdominal breathing. Just let it be easy and relaxed.

As you relax, gradually allow yourself to breathe more slowly.

Start to let a little more time pass after you exhale and before you inhale again. It doesn't matter if the size of your breaths is irregular. You may begin to feel sleepy, but don't let yourself fall asleep before you've completed the exercise.

Keeping relaxed and focused, remain aware of the rate of your breathing and let it slow down. After two to five minutes, let your breathing slow down again and begin to concentrate on your heartbeat. Get a sense of your heart's rate of contraction, but don't actually count your heartbeats because doing that will interfere with your relaxation. Just notice each beat and generally be aware of the pace. Once you get a steady feeling, think about letting your heart slow down and just form the idea without any expectation of time frame.

You will feel yourself breathing more deeply and your heart slowing down even more. Slowly and comfortably instruct your heart to go even slower as you lead it into more and more relaxed rhythms. The tension will release from your body as you do this. Maintain this slow steady state for as long as you like, and, when you're finished, you can, if you want, fall asleep.

The next exercise will also help many people for whom discomfort or anger fuels the need to eat and overeat.

The Anger-Releasing Exercise

Although some researchers would say that anger-releasing methods such as punching a pillow only lead to the creation of more anger, I believe that this is not necessarily true. So many people have built-up anger that once they tap into it and release it, it feels good to release even more. While I certainly don't recommend hitting people or surrounding yourself with angry people or hostile circumstances, I do believe in the absolute value of releasing this damaging emotional energy. The exercise can take anywhere from five minutes to one hour. After completing the exercise, it would be a good idea to augment its benefits by engaging in some positive self-talk, and repeating affirmations of joy.

It's also a good idea to take a close look at why you've built up all this anger. You don't want to wind up punching the pillow so routinely that you have no place left to put your head down. And expressing your anger at a person or a problem may be only a temporary solution. You might really need to change a situation or change whatever it is in you that's causing you to allow it to happen.

Our minds tend to imagine and then manifest situations that allow us to expend our built-up anger, so that the angrier we are, the more negative we become. The result isn't relief, but more bad outcomes, frustration, and missed opportunities brought into our lives. That said, at some time, every one of us is going to find him- or herself at the bottom of the pecking order, being dumped, or picked on by too many people. When that happens, you effectively have no one on whom to expend your own accumulated anger and, typically, keep it inside. All that negative energy in your body acts like a toxic substance.

Our society generally disapproves of anger, causing us to "stuff down" our emotions instead of expressing them. If you're in that position, it wouldn't be unusual for you to try to counter all that negativity with the "safe" pleasure of overeating or engaging in other so-called safe but actually harmful activities.

This exercise, then, will be extremely useful for getting rid of anger carried over from the past. If, for example, someone hurt you or wronged you and that person is no longer around, you can still act out your hostility privately and productively. You can still tell that person off, and if it gives you relief, you may even forgive and forget.

Before we begin, a word of caution: Because this exercise asks you to be very vocal, don't do it in a place or at a time when your yelling can disturb anyone else. Find someplace private and do one or more of the following things: Imagine the person you're angry at in the room with you. Yell at him or her loudly and with your full diaphragm. Shake your fists. Kick and shout. I also recommend punching a pillow. Make sure it's big and sturdy enough to take a good punch and made of a material that won't hurt your hands. Punch it, kick it, step on it, while telling it every angry thing you need to get out.

You might not even be angry at a specific person. Maybe you're just angry with life or with the world. Shake your fists and allow yourself to do whatever it is that will release your anger and make you feel like you've dumped your emotional load. Afterwards, you'll feel very relaxed.

The Giant Will Stomping Exercise

This exercise will help you to assert your will in a resistant world. Use it when you make a plan but find it difficult to implement or when you need to affirm your perspective in a difficult situation. Use it to affirm something positive about yourself. It is a version of an exercise from Lee Lipsenthal MD., who is a past president of the American Board of Holistic Medicine.

If you're easy-going and generally find it difficult to speak up for yourself, you will find this exercise particularly beneficial. It helps you to connect your body to your mental energy so that your physical and emotional selves are in alignment with your purpose. Your will is, therefore, magnified. The exercise will take from five to 20 minutes.

Find a private space, preferably with a wood or carpeted floor. Think of a statement you need to affirm or own as the truth. It might be, "Yes, I am free!" or, "No! Don't tell me what to do, or "Yes! I can do it!" Do this exercise with the more positively-stated situations. Imagine that you are a giant as you say or shout the words. Make your statement assertively physical by stomping on the floor for emphasis. Don't hurt yourself. Move slowly and thump like a giant.

As you shout, use your arms to get your entire body into it. Move around the room. Keep shouting and stomping on the floor with each word. Fling your arms into the air. This is sort of a magnified tai chi exercise that moves you from thought to action by integrating your physical and emotional self with your mental self.

The following exercise increases your sense of pleasure.

The Expression of Love Exercise

This is an exercise in sensuality that allows you to communicate intimately with the world around you. It increases the ability to express joy and emotions. Sensuality relaxes the borders and defensive walls we normally put up between and around ourselves in the course of everyday life. It is a way for us to let go of the emotional control we exert on how others can touch us and how we express ourselves in return.

Sensuality can occur between you and another person or between you and a rock or a pet or a piece of art. It's a natural way to give and receive the love we all seek in our lives. The exercise is a safe and joyful way to develop your awareness of all that is "non-you," to help you express your vulnerability and open yourself up to receiving love. Take as long as you want with it and repeat it often.

You need to find a private room or outdoor space to do the exercise. Go around to every object in the space you've chosen and verbally express your love while touching the object. If you like, you can express your love in your thoughts without speaking it out loud, but be sure that you feel it throughout your body. Be sincere. As with all of life, it's what's in your heart that matters. When you do the exercise with living plants and trees, don't be surprised if you feel that you've heard them reply.

This next exercise is an especially important one:

The Self-Loving Exercise

This exercise is designed to communicate your love for yourself to your mind through its hard-wired connections with your body. It will fill you with the love that you may have been lacking in your life. Simply acknowledging a part of your body that needs love may bring up memories of an emotional injury that occurred long ago. If you feel resistance, you can do a "contemplation" or use the Age Count-Back Exercise I describe later to uncover the original cause of the block. You may need to repeat the exercise many times because you are dealing with your entire lifetime. It should take from five to 45 minutes.

Lie down or sit comfortably in a chair. Your eyes can be open or closed. Slowly touch every part of your body and as you do, tell yourself that you love you. *Feel* happiness and joy. Speak the words aloud or just say them to yourself. As you touch each part, name it: "I love you, feet." "I love my legs," and so on. By doing this, you affirm your affection for all of yourself, bring balance to your entire being and resolve conflicts within your body.

Often, old negative, imprinted emotions will be stuck in or associated with particular parts of your body. Touching those parts will often reveal the block or negativity associated with something in your past. You need to release and change these negative associations and replace them with self-acceptance and understanding of your own unique beauty so you can be free from illness and live the best life you can. Any part of your body that resists allowing itself to be loved deserves contemplation. Many illnesses result from a lack of self-love, which can sometimes be physically isolated in your body.

A variation on this exercise would be to give yourself an oil or lotion massage, feeling love for yourself and all parts of your body as you do the massage. This promotes sensuality, a quality from which many of us have grown detached.

This inner emotional exercise that follows is useful when you need security and need to stabilize unwanted tension and stress in your emotional body. It fosters balance and peace. I use this one frequently.

The Color Absorption Exercise

Different wavelengths of light actually have different color properties, and when you bring color into your body, it will help balance your inner state. You may, for example, find that you want to eat different fruits and vegetables on different days, depending upon their color. There are overlapping applications of energy that exist among the nutrition, color, and energy needs of your body and spirit. This is a new awareness for some people. You'll find that you need to bring in a certain color for a different length of time on different days. You can even make preferences by color throughout your day to create balance within yourself. The exercise takes between 8 and 15 minutes to complete.

Find a comfortable position and close your eyes. One by one, imagine each color of the rainbow (red, orange, yellow, green, blue, purple, then violet)—as well as black and white, if you wish. First, consider the color, then take it into your mind so that you "see" it internally. Feel yourself pulling the color into your body, to the core of your being, in every cell, more and more with every breath. As you do this, you will know when you've soaked enough into yourself.

You can do anger dumping exercises occasionally. You can do pleasure exercises and peaceful meditation exercises frequently. You have to release the unfulfilled emotional drives in a state of openness, reception and love. You will be filled up with lasting peace eventually. You have to go beyond the thinking past of your brain to engage emotional realities to assemble your life back together in peace, joy and contentment to have the emotional power of stability.

Re-inventing your life emotionally is one of the foundations of a healthy body. You will have new goals of true health—that's for sure. New drives engaging your body and emotions with joy and sustainable pleasure, a must! For just about everyone, this will mean a slowing down of how you experience life. A rushed life without adequate intake of real joy will run you out of emotional fuel. Depression and excess physical weight can result. The slowing down of experiences to allow emotional contact and reality to come into us will begin to satisfy and stabilize your true needs and life drives.

Your mental concepts will be altered as they are connected to your emotional drives. Old drives will dissipate. Emotional capability will expand. Love fosters your growth and maintains it. This takes time and by now you have started to realize that the whole sense of time, as you've lived it before, must be thrown away to "no sense of time." That is, it is a process that has no limits of how long you will continue to improve yourself.

You're beginning to experience life new, throwing away old concepts, slowing down and opening up the feeling of love and contentment which is a sustainable form of pleasure. You change from false ill health to true health. You change from "poor me," to "how can I help you." Whether you know it or not in the beginning, you will have developed true intelligence. Accept the unexpected as part of a better genuine life. "Cookies" will mean nothing and the drive for empty rewards will lessen and eventually disappear. Life is sustainable as it should be. We are more than our bodies, and our bodies can become a path to our true spirit.

If you have accumulated anxiety, anger, unexpressed traumatic energy, you won't go to the light, you'll be driven to darkness and conflict

Deal with the original cause and the light will not shine any straighter

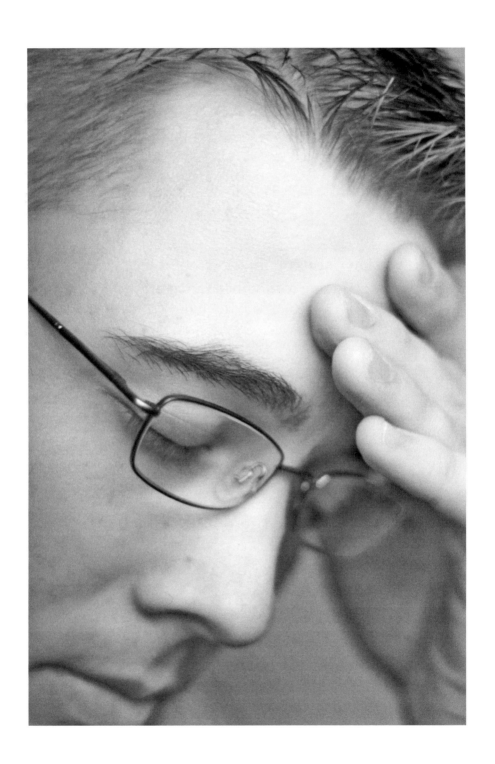

Chapter Five

Losing the Mental Weight

Your Thoughts

Your beliefs are a more controlling level of personal consciousness than your emotions and cause you to direct your drives and emotions. They generate and define the emotions and feelings you have when you interact in the world around you and we call that "attitude." They must be considered very important when you are trying to lose weight because it is inevitable that your very thoughts are traced back to the origin of why you are overweight.

Examples of thoughts that can relate to pathological eating for pleasure are these: If you don't believe you deserve pleasure or social interaction you won't seek out either one. Then because you have inherent human needs for companionship and social interaction, you tend to compensate for this lack of pleasure of being with others by overeating both in frequency and quantity. Often this will be towards the end of the day between 4:30 p.m. and 2 a.m. when the drives are most built up and unsatisfied.

Perception is not the same truth for all of us. For example, if you go into a room, you might look out a window and see a beautiful bird on a branch. The scene makes you feel good and you have a positive sensation, a joy. Another person might look out that same window and want to shoo the bird away and then focus on a distant gray cloud and worry whether or not it will bring a cold wind with it. Not a joyful response, but one of frustration, maybe boredom, maybe bitterness. People are different. Your perspective is important. Being positive is very important for shaping your future. Many people think ahead and project negative outcomes in life in order to emotionally protect themselves in a preemptive way. These imagined ideas of how things will turn out, however, rarely happen. Depression is an example of preemptive protected thinking for some people.

Consider these important steps:

Pinpoint the inner thoughts that limit you or generate negative emotions. From a few deeply held beliefs, you generate most of your drives and subsequent emotions. Any belief that is negative to your self or views of others or the world tends to lower your energy. Fearful beliefs about anything, including yourself, tend to generate higher agitation energies. By finding your beliefs you find your blocks; you can work with the techniques that enable you to identify your sources of defeat. Your mind and emotions will no longer be unfamiliar and uncontrollable areas of mystery.

If you find opposition to this mindful approach, you need to look to your thinking patterns and self beliefs that have drawn a curtain down on your feelings and vulnerability. The typical histories that cause this are about traumatic events in the past that cause you to emotionally block yourself from feeling at all. You can use the "Age Count-Back Exercise" on page 80 which also first appeared in my book, *Start Living Stop Dying – 10 Steps to Natural Health*, to find what originally triggered such events in your life and when you started limiting your emotional self.

The answer for you could be beliefs and conclusions you've made about yourself that say, for example, you don't deserve love. When this happens, you won't generate enough positive feelings spontaneously or from the interactions you have in life. This is a faulty belief that resides in many people leading to a type of emotional overeating. Whether you know it or not, do it or not, your core drives of life will compel you to pleasure–so you can eat it or live it.

Healthy thoughts lead to healthy feelings which lead to a healthy body and a weight that's right for you. *The Inside-Outside Diet* shows that **losing weight by purely physical means, that is, drugs or quick weight-loss or gimmicky diets—is a ridiculous concept that has no good consequences over the long term.**

Being active is a key concept in your belief system because being active is what your body does *not* become as your mind becomes more affected by harmful beliefs. Harmful beliefs and habits paralyze you. Has this, for example, happened to you? You see someone you want to know, but your beliefs about who you are and who that person might be charge negative emotions instead. You're sure you'll be rejected! You feel the "loss" from your own negative self beliefs that got you "rejected" before you even made a move. If you start to manufacture negative energies, that other person might even "pick up" on your very thoughts unconsciously and be turned off by you before you even speak a word or look at them. Negative self-beliefs do damage to your true health and body. Excess weight is just one of the possible outcomes. Have for example, harmful beliefs and habits paralyzed your motivation to exercise?

Your inner reality consists of your thoughts and beliefs that play on your feelings on a daily basis. These thoughts, in turn, power the feelings that drive you to action, inaction or wrong action. Eating pounds of sugar and drinking gallons of coffee would be wrong actions to take to compensate for an unsatisfied, un-pleasurable and tense inner life. Corporations have made tons of money based on your need for compensatory pleasure as a means to release tension. When you don't fulfill your emotional needs directly, you end up with a greater desire for entertainment. That is exactly what you have going on in the United States now as people seek ways to be entertained. Instead of entertainment being a distraction from stress relief and boredom, entertainment should primarily be a route for creativity, social sharing and interaction. Entertainment should be a pleasure and not just an unconscious tension release.

Now you may say you eat because you're nervous or bored, but those "feelings" are generated by your beliefs combined with what you tell yourself is true. For example, if you tell yourself you're ugly and unwanted, you will feel depressed and become asocial while your need for feeling accepted for yourself and feel pleasure may come from dipping heavily into the ice cream. You've heard people say, "Food is my friend," and they make it so. True emotional balance isn't found in fat and sugar. Positive thinking alone will probably not be enough to correct this kind of deeply-rooted belief. If this is you, you may need to directly examine your past.

Caffeine is a stimulant that weakens your natural willpower

Coffee shops have sprung up everywhere in the United States and cater to personal and societal stress by promising that pleasure in a cup will temporarily cure your problems. In fact, caffeine may be partly responsible for many illnesses. **Caffeine increases blood pressure in susceptible people and leads to reciprocal fatigue. Caffeine antagonizes atrial fibrillation and leads to insomnia.** Caffeine is a stimulant that alters neurohormonal balance. It temporarily boosts awareness while over-stimulating the body. Caffeine effectively undermines your true willpower and energy.

Caffeine is a semi-powerful, mind-affecting drug. It is a "perfect" addictive drug in that it alters how you mentally and emotionally function without totally incapacitating you from performance at work. I believe it is very harmful and one of the greatest contributors of continuing stress and social disease in western culture. Coffee, anxiety, stress and sugar consumption are tied very closely to the obesity epidemic in the United States.

When you're sleeping, you have active thoughts and beliefs that dictate your next move, your next choices, your abilities and capabilities and all the emotions that come from your interaction with others in the environment. Beliefs can be unconscious because they were instilled from infancy into your memory.

If you believe you are alone in the world and that you will not survive, you will function with tension as the overriding drive in influencing every little thing you do. That anxiety will never give you peace but only lead to inner and outer unrest. That unrest may lead to compulsions, obsessions, and greater tension, all of which drive you right into the primary bad choice you make for the imbalance: overeating. As you see, it's not unusual for disease to follow. These beliefs can be from 10, 20 or 30 years ago and not be in your waking memory. Hypnotherapy may be useful in helping you to remember early incidents in your past that are affecting you now. If you feel deeply blocked or unable to get improvements from your own contemplations, consider receiving outside help from psychologists, therapists or sometimes hypnotherapists.

Beliefs can be powerful, and most of us fight for what we believe is the truth. Some of us not only want that truth to be valid, but want others to agree with us, even if it's not right for you or for them at all. If you are a person who has to be right, then you may engage in too many unnecessary conflicts that provoke stress. Stress as we know can lead to overeating.

If you have a fear of poverty or of losing what makes you feel secure or worry too much about money, then your stress level will climb. In fact, almost any belief based on fear or negative outcome will affect you emotionally and either limit your emotional growth or cause the discomfort of stress. I mention these specific beliefs because they often underlie superficial stress and overeating.

The modern day person's mind is very busy. There are so many choices and decisions to consider and act upon. If your inner beliefs are that "you have to be right," or that "you can't make a mistake because your life value is at stake," then all the numerous choices in the world will greatly stress you, even if those decisions are really trivial. Even going to the grocery store may raise your stress energy. Correcting that underlying belief would then be curative.

The mind also doesn't like time with nothing to do--a factor that greatly affects people who run their lives by their watches. This gives rise to another commonly-held belief that there are no minutes within 24 hours for exercise. If this sounds like you, the belief is based on your perception of exercise which is that you haven't the time, and that exercising, therefore, is a waste of time.

Financial beliefs cause many distressful life choices. A client told me that she won't give up working for $9 an hour at a stressful job and, therefore, turned down an offer of a similar job at a non-stressful workplace for $8 hour, starting pay, where she may have a better chance for advancement. Or, I'm sure we all know someone who earns $290,000 a year at a difficult job, and is there for the money, instead of making $120,000 a year at a job they'd love immensely and not risk having a heart attack.

Why do they do as they do? It could be social and cultural shaping, out-of-control competitive drives to earn more, or a concern for financially securing the future and allaying retirement fears, which may never be realized. Both the $9 an hour worker and the $290,000 go-getter, do not even consider physical health, and believe that the calories they expend on the job is as good as exercising. Their priorities will never achieve for them a healthy weight or life –unless they consciously decide to re-prioritize what their life is about.

Not only do you need to set into motion a life-changing clean-up of your beliefs to have a healthy body weight, but you need to go full throttle with positive affirmations about yourself - including exercise as being important and fun to do. This is a bit of self-administered brainwashing, but it helps you begin to counteract the negative beliefs that the culture has already "fed" you. You must deliberately examine your choices when it comes to altering your lifestyle to be healthier.

If your thoughts are run by tension or boredom, eating temporarily takes that sensation away. You're feeding your problems and temporarily numbing them. But the mind is persistent. Whatever was going on in your mind resurfaces after eating *because your mind is originally generating it. Original anxiety, original tension, original boredom will self-propagate again and again, if only because thoughts are empowered from the inside out.*

Harmful beliefs paralyze you from taking meaningful action to improve your life

"You are what you eat" is not quite as accurate a statement as the more truthful, "you are what you think." If you are depressed, your body will show it. If you are nervous and tense, your body will show that too. If you think you don't deserve to be loved, your behavior will reflect it and others can pick up those signals. If you think you won't succeed at anything, you probably won't do anything or find ways to undermine your own progress.

However, if you think eating is fun and that it's the only fun you've ventured out for in the last 20 years, then you'll probably keep overeating. You're stuck believing it is the only way you can enjoy yourself. This is what your mind is pulling out of its repetitive short term memory. It takes many repetitions of good new choices to eventually replace your old memories.

It helps to remember that the mind operates on a circuitry, so to speak, and is like a computerized program that takes in data and continues to bring to fruition the thought it is running at the time. Add a negative thought about your self-esteem (for example, "My husband is right. I can't handle the kids."), and your mental computer will run and rerun the thought. Soon, the thought is ingrained and part of you, manifesting itself in real life, getting you to be sure not to manage the kids effectively, while you don't know why it's happening. Weren't you trying? Yes and no. What you did was make yourself fail. This is why it is so important to know what your thoughts are and clean them up. **This is your responsibility and no one else can do it for you.**

When you were young, your parents and peers all contributed to who you became and how you changed. You need to go beyond those influences and take care of your own clean-up. If you have children, your supreme responsibility is to live the best you can–*when you know what that is!*

Your Memory

I've brought up the subject of short-term memory a number of times, and want you to understand in more detail why it is so important. I need to emphasize this: How you respond to stress is usually simply patterned after what your parents did to handle it. It's that short-term memory that continually draws out how we habitually act to cope and satisfy current emotional situations. Finding and fixing any non-serving beliefs from your past may be key to your personal revelation of the cure for your overweight condition. Using the techniques of contemplation and the "Age Count-Back Exercise" described later, you can track down and relinquish the detrimental emotional imprints and memories from your past that may be at the heart of your being overweight. But also know that you can't stay thinking about the past; you have to move to the present to be in the "now" of correct living and bring your awareness to the present.

Your short-term memory is like an index card catalog of experiences, feelings and thoughts your body goes to when it needs a solution to anything. Let's say that you are overweight because you overeat. Your mind probably holds 300 to 1000 bits of short-term memory experiences, say, including one where you indulged in a chocolate sundae as a means of pleasure. You actually stored it in your mind and labeled it 300 to 1000 times as "delicious" "comforting" and "positive" when in actuality, it was damaging you. That sundae redirected your physical energy--and you probably first got a sugar high

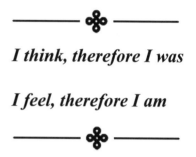

I think, therefore I was

I feel, therefore I am

before crashing and then "needing" more sugar. It took your energy away from conscious mental acuity and it might have even fueled a mild allergic response. What's sure about the sundae is that it contributed to your being overweight and clouded your road to recovery. It set in pattern a problem-solution response that your mind hung on to for physical emotional relief. That can't remain in you for you to be healthy, but it will take a year of memory replacement to change this response to healthier ones. That is why you have to be patient and persistent.

You have many short-term memory habits like this one that reinforce the patterns you create every time you think or feel or act a certain way. Your body goes to its memory base of responses. If you have a weight problem, you need to change these patterns. Start now, because it takes time to replace old undermining memories with new self-affirming habits.

This story sharpens the point. I had a friend who took a temporary job at an office where the environment was a bit anxious. The acceptable office culture was to take a break at an in-house coffee establishment where everyone let their hair down for up to 15 minutes. Though he planned on being at this job only two months, it stretched to four months. The problem was that he succumbed to the coffee-and-donut-letting-it-all-out daily practice. He started to put on nearly 10 pounds of extra abdominal weight, even though he had been thin his entire life. He knew he had to pull himself out of that donut hole and change his eating habits at the office.

Before he quit this job, he started to bring his own apples and bananas to work with two healthy water bottles that he kept in a small container. He began to confront the belief that the donut was good. He started his own counter-strategy to the office norm before leaving and received some kidding for bringing his own snacks. Interestingly, a few other people started doing similarly healthy meal preparations at the job before he ended up leaving.

Even small things you do can be helpful just as small bad habits can be detrimental in the long run, too. It also shows what may be going on in your home relative to what you do and what your children may be learning. Do the right thing at home, too, because you are setting an example and implanting within your children all your best and worst traits, whether you know it or not.

Right here is one element to why food diets don't work: **you'd still be operating from old automatic responses from your short-term memory that continue to strengthen your connection to food being the solution**. Counting calories and increasing your brain time spent on food eventually results in eating all those food thoughts in real life later. Depending upon your body genetics, your body will then make fat at the rate of your calorie consumption.

Continue to put yourself on a course of change with these steps:

*Correct your opinions of yourself if they get in the way of emotional growth.

*Get on with your dream or true desires, enthusiasm and joy.

*Resolve the drives that waste your time and make you unhealthy.

*Simplify your true wants. You will actually start to feel more compassion and express positive feelings with patience. This will slow you down and make you more effective at what you apply yourself to do. This will show that you're able to create balance inside you, which eliminates anxiety and promotes peace, security and health.

How to Change Your Thoughts

When I say, "mental weight," I'm referring to the burdens you bring to what you think. If you think everyone hates you and it doesn't really matter to you, that isn't a burden. If you think everyone loves you and you can't stand the responsibility of give-and-take, then that is a burden.

Thinking does not in itself necessarily give joy–thinking detracts from joy or any emotion really. Awareness is joy. Thinking however, is the governor of what your emotions become. *Mental weight* has an important role in weight loss. Self-beliefs are frequently the ultimate target of anyone wanting to correct their emotional drives which lead to overeating and excess weight. Your beliefs can be altered and this is something modern medicine hasn't wanted to tackle for it involves invisible turf that has never been adequately defined in modern society. But there are techniques when you know the reality. That said, no physician or therapist will ever be able to change you – only you can do that.

Changing your thoughts is possible in several ways. First, you can rethink and *re-label* all your memories related to food in the past, and pinpoint the food memories that you called good and now you know are actually bad. Re-labeling old memories about food that has done you no good should be captioned--for example, calling that chocolate sundae something like "high-cal compost" so that your desire for it will diminish. This might seem simple but the mind works on basic principles.

Next, educate yourself as to what foods are better for you. Remind yourself of what foods are good versus bad the next time you feel stressed, bored or in need of security and can sense that you are about to let a bad food memory take you over. Then eat something light and healthful or go for a walk. Everyone who is overweight needs to be educated about what foods help and which do not. The *Holistic Nutrition* section that follows, reveals more about what these good foods are.

Next, when you feel stressed or bored, make new experiences or choices, find new directions and build a new plan not based on old short-term memory dictates. A pre-made plan helps you create new memory experiences. If you turned to chocolate ice cream and whipped cream for comfort in the past, choose kiwi or carrots now and keep them in your frig. You can't eat the healthier foods if you don't stock them in your home. Walk around the block. Keep your shoes by the door. Help someone who's housebound and go outside yourself. Snack only on healthful foods. Keep Brazil nuts and almonds in jars on the kitchen counter for protein snacks. Many small changes will have their effect.

These newly created experiences will, in time, outweigh negative urges and be more influential than your old concepts and patterns. This is why it takes a year to implement change. You have to create these new responses and be sure to label them "healthy" and good. The more repetitions you get in, the stronger they will grow.

It is OK if you go back every so often to old foods. But you will find that this happens less and less frequently until your old responses are eliminated from short-term memory storage as the choice behind your overeating. Furthermore, when you do try old foods, you slowly experience with clarity the negative effects of certain foods on your body. You won't like the lack of control or distracting emotions you feel because of them. For example, you won't like the jitters you get from coffee or the dullness you get from a chocolate bar. Often, after you have made a switch to natural foods, eating old processed foods make you feel terrible. So even if you go back to an old habit, you are likely to benefit from the negative experience.

One technique to reinforce change of emotions and the thoughts that underlie them is by using Bach flower remedies. Bach flower essences are harvested from specific flowers that are said to have the effect of altering your subtle energies and emotions. Personally, I have found Bach flower remedies to be like homeopathic medicine which work best on sensitive people on an energetic frequency level. I use the flower essences in a specific way. Each 20cc bottle of the 38 Bach flower remedies has written on the label the effect the flower essence is supposed to have.

For those who would like to use this technique, I suggest you read the label before applying the essence under your tongue. In this way, the user reinforces in their mind the changes they are wishing to create. For example, those needing to lower stress energy may use the "Rescue" remedy or rock rose. Reading the rock rose essence label, one would say to themselves, this flower remedy "adds courage and presence of mind in the face of terror or extreme fear." For those needing to raise their energy from being too low, try the essences of rock water or wild rose. Each bottle will have a written affirmation that you can use to reinforce upon your consciousness the energy change you would like to have. This is a technique that can be calming for stressful people or uplifting for those with low energy. Give this technique a try if you feel this combination of flower remedies and self-talk will help you reinforce change in your emotional and mental disposition.

Both boredom and stress can lead to *mindless eating*—the food is there and you keep at it, stoking it in, not really tasting it, while talking to others or watching TV. Because you have numbed your body from the negative feelings you are currently experiencing, it takes a lot of food eating to break through and make you feel better. Be aware of what is happening if this is you. Make a plan that will help you redirect stress and boredom issues to non-eating fulfillment.

One step you can take is to make a list of your overeating habits and then list what you could do instead of eating at that time of day. In the beginning, keep a journal of your overeating episodes and you will start to see a pattern of reactionary eating.

Keeping a journal keeps you honest

These episodes will give you the foresight to plan other remedies when you feel the kind of discomfort that leads to such overeating. What you are doing is empowering yourself by becoming knowledgeable of what makes you tick. **One reason there are so many illnesses in the west is because western culture has never included mental self-knowledge as part of a healthy cultural lifestyle.**

I need to re-emphasize these points for you to help you succeed: You can recall your day by using the technique of contemplation to remember the feeling you had prior to wanting to eat. Contemplate what circumstances preceded your impulse to eat. Search for the root of the issue by asking yourself *why* you have a certain thought or feeling. Keep asking the question until you get no further answers to the *why*. Make a list of your fears and you will often see your belief limitations emerge. *Understand what you are changing from, and who you are changing into -a much healthier, wiser person.* Often it is very useful to see yourself as an "old" you and a "new" you. Which choice do you want now? Who is running your life now? What does the new you want to do?

Another technique to make a change is to actively confirm new beliefs daily through self affirmations. This daily work helps implant a belief system you can then function by. Remember: *You need to reinforce new beliefs for one year to make them strong. Say them five times a day and five times a week for 30 weeks. Actualize them through some sort of action three times a week for 20 weeks and they will be even stronger.* This will strengthen your new short-term memory by replacing old poor choices with new proactive solutions.

Many of your drives boil down to a *few specific beliefs* or thoughts that underlie them that have managed to run your relationship with food. You have a finite number of core drives guiding your life--the list isn't endless. Think of the beliefs you encounter within you as rocks you carry on your back in a knapsack. Identifying them, making them smaller or just getting rid of them will lighten your load and your body. No one wants to go hiking with an overburdened backpack of weight.

A technique that works to find the harmful beliefs is the reliable "time-line" approach to determine when you became an overeater and overweight. Take a look back. What conclusions did you make early in your life that started the chain of harmful overeating. These questions can get you started:

*When did the excess poundage first go on?

*If you are unhappy, when did you stop being happy?

*When did you start living a stressful life?

*When did you give up your dreams?

*When did you start making food a conscious means of enjoyment in your life?

*When were you last at a normal and healthful weight?

*What was your life like when you had no weight problems?

*Finally, if you could remake your life, what would it be like and what would you be doing?

Use the "Age Count-Back Exercise," coming up next, to figure out what was going on at the time harmful emotional traits originated. This may be a key for you to uncover and change bad patterns left over from your past. Because I can't predict what you, the reader, have specifically in your mind as limiting beliefs, I have given many examples. The fact that you must have specific beliefs originating your drives is incontrovertible.

The Age Count-Back Exercise

This age-related memory exercise enhances the self-discoveries you've made through contemplation. It will help you determine when you made a significant change in the way you think, and what happened to you at an early age that significantly affected your life.

This exercise takes from 15-45 minutes. It asks you to count backwards from your age now, but it can also be done in reverse, counting forward from some specific younger age to where you are now.

Some of your opinions about your own worth, your abilities, intelligence, and courage have been created at various times in your life. It's therefore useful, when you do this exercise, to focus on some specific belief or feeling whose origin you want to discover. Continue the same way for as many beliefs as you would like to uncover, clarify and change.

Let's begin:

*To start, find a comfortable position, preferably, lying down. Close your eyes and recall your life as of this month. Describe aloud or to yourself how you feel and what's going on. Then do the same for the previous year. For example, your self dialogue might be, "It's 2008 and I'm working at a job I don't like. I'm seeing Cathy (or Mike) and it's going alright, but I have to admit that our relationship suffers because I'm so negative and critical."

*Keep going back, year by year, as far as you need to go. As you continue to do this, eventually you'll come to a time--probably during your youth--when you didn't act or feel the way you are now. At that point, hone in on the time of year, the month, even the day if you can, and start to recall specific events. The triggering event may have been obviously traumatic, such as the death of a loved one, or it may be something that is apparently innocuous and unimportant. However big or small, it doesn't matter. What matters is how it affected you.

Recall how you felt and also, how you coped.

*Keep remembering and you will usually uncover events, people, and circumstances that you know are linked to your current beliefs or behaviors. When you get to the specifics, that defining moment, you will probably understand that you misinterpreted an event, a word, an attitude that made you feel belittled or inadequate or unwanted--something that led to the way you are now.

*Once you've gotten to the source event and visual memory of an old harmful belief, you can understand how it was implanted. Then you can change that belief more effectively. Powerful emotional events may even discharge themselves from your body at this time of discovery. Begin by telling yourself that you (or others) made a mistake, that your feelings have changed, and that you want to be different. You want and deserve to be happy. You want to notice and validate positive qualities in others. And because you want to be happy, you will focus on projecting images of a positive future. You will know that if something doesn't work out, you'll still be okay. Bad things often happen as a means to change. You talk to the old belief in a way that most reverses it and proves it wrong in your mind.

*Do this exercise until you feel sure you've captured the defining moments that made your beliefs so damaging and food so important.

Your weight is an exact reflection of your inner mental state and resultant emotional blueprint. Your body has simply been following your own inner directions of what you've become. As you interpret the world around you differently, you will start to emit happy emotions and a light body. All this occurs by changing your controlling beliefs.

Understanding this hierarchal power of how your inner beliefs eventually result in the drives, choices and emotions that you create is fundamental to altering your body for optimal health.

You might not be aware or conscious of what your inner choices are now, but if you want to change, the first key is *self awareness*. Part of that awareness is knowing that your choices are made by *both outside and inside influences*.

Patients have told me about wanting to "fit in" with a certain crowd, who make eating take-out junk food a big part of socializing--the more junk, the better. Other patients say they know that they should not be digging in to five candy bars, and ignore the warnings from voices in their heads that say, "toss it, don't touch it." Unfortunately, they relent with defeatist thinking, "I'll never get my body in shape so what's the difference?" Or they subconsciously say, "I'm going to do *something* nice for me today."

Unless you become *aware* of what you're feeling and doing, your healthier *outside* food choices will not take hold. Your old internal dictates will continue to manifest the body you have and the unhealthy way of life that are currently programmed within you. What you want is for new programming to guide you, or those old outside images and influences will continue to manipulate your entire life. Change the programming and you change the result. While healthier food and bodily drives can heal your feelings, it is by far more permanent to *cure yourself from the Inside-out*.

You see the world through your eyes and project your inner thoughts and beliefs onto the world to determine what's going on around you--and in how others see you. Because the world is filtered through your very subjective views, how you talk to yourself is extremely important. This is why getting to the source of your old beliefs is so important: you see which judgments you've proved wrong and can be tossed out. Then you can affirm the new beliefs to your deepest core.

To reinforce your new, positive feelings and perspectives, find a tangible reminder that you can look at throughout the day. For example, you could buy a butterfly key chain because the butterfly is a symbol of joy and freedom. Or maybe you'd prefer a dragonfly, which symbolizes change. Eventually, you'll no longer need reminders or physical things to reinforce your new outlook on yourself and your life. Every little bit helps in the beginning.

<u>Why You Feel Anxiety or Stress</u>

When you encounter a stressful environmental source (say, your job or daily trials of survival) you have two choices: One, you can eliminate, avoid or deny the environmental event, hoping, that you don't encounter it again or, more beneficially, you can decide to change the internal trigger that leads you to believe you are in jeopardy or in a serious conflict of survival. While there are real dangers to life, some of the stress we feel is meant to protect us from harm if we are threatened. It is useful to know when to stop being preoccupied with fears about survival so you can allow outright change to occur, versus health-damaging worry

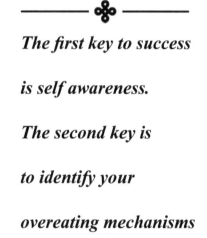

The first key to success is self awareness. The second key is to identify your overeating mechanisms

that causes no improvement, but instead, creates ill health. As has been said by many people, what you can affect, *do*, what you cannot control, stop worrying and let it go.

Not counting real disasters—you get fired or the bank threatens to foreclose, most worries are exaggerated fears and concerns that never really actualize. Knowing this can be comforting. Sometimes it will be obvious that your worrisome belief is false, that is, there is really no evidence to prove the event will happen. These worries weigh you down and can drive you to chips, fries or that gallon of nut fudge ice cream for comfort. Stop the reaction by first pre-emptively striking the worry from your being!

Eliminate the belief that generates emotional anxiety and elevates stress to a persistent nervous energy. That energy can over stimulate your adrenal glands, which results in more adrenaline or cortisol pumping into your system. It is that constant hormonal release that you feel as stress that eventually leads to emotional exhaustion as revealed in depression and physical fatigue. Early high energy stress releases both cortisol and dopamine to prepare us for action and insult. Later, "burnt out" stress leads to a hypo-functioning depression with low levels of both neurohormones: cortisol and dopamine, making you feel worse.

You can't focus on being productive and actualizing your goals when your life is about escaping anxiety, despair and depression, all of which result from your having chronic stressful thoughts. As a doctor, I know the power that changed thinking holds for you in curing your overeating problems.

Contemplation can again be used to eliminate stressful thoughts. Through contemplation, you can actually "hear" your own mind generate the thoughts that it does and get an understanding for how your mind functions. Your motivation may have started with wanting to lose weight, but you may end up on the psychological level of dealing with your core life beliefs that have far more beneficial impact on your life and health than just your weight. The truth is that to be different, you're going to have to be different in your lifestyle, how you think and generate emotions. Lip service to change will not magically be implemented in your life, rather, you must take action and reinforce the new beliefs over time.

For example: You can hear yourself say things like, "I've had it, I'm too old, too unhealthy," or, "I'm losing control, even worse than before," or " I'm too frustrated about watching what I eat—what's the difference, anyway," or, "I can't stop myself eating sugar, but if I don't, I know I'll die," or whatever is important to you. Now turn the negative thought into a positive one and state it within yourself by flipping it. It will sound like, "I want to have a healthy body, and I want to be happy," or, "I want to know how to gain control of my body and my life," and so on. Later, "I want to" will become "I am."

When you contemplate, you must consider only *one* issue at a time and follow it back. It's best to deal with only one question a day to give yourself a chance to tap into that self-knowledge. Too many tasks will increase the chance that you'll be distracted from fully completing any one contemplative goal.

Using the *Inside-Outside* techniques, change can start here: Contemplate why you overeat and why you are overweight. Is it about not exercising? If so, why aren't you exercising? Is it about not being able to stop eating from dinner time to bedtime? What's happening to you then? Keep asking yourself the questions that are pertinent to you.

I suggest that you write down your questions and your immediate answers and realizations, and then go back and review them. Use a checklist to be sure you answer all your questions or issues completely to their origin.

To help get more effective results, you need to start thinking, "is this good for me?" instead of, "does that taste good!" *How you phrase things in your mind is important.* Feel good about that which makes you healthy, capable and fit. You need to feel secure from your own intentional emotional generation and not falsely stimulate those feelings through coffee, donuts, steak, potatoes and pasta.

The new thoughts you implant in your mind should reflect constructive beliefs, such as "less food is more" and "no dessert is healthier." If you're a fast-food fan because you rely on the "I don't want to wait" mentality, contemplate what this means to you. Why the urgency about getting food? Why do you only buy the cheapest products when they are often the most unhealthy? Whatever undermining emotions run this program in you, it must be removed. Instead, learn to give yourself time to enjoy eating intentionally, and know that there will always be enough food out there for you. Simplicity and patience will almost always serve your life better.

In fact, you will get more pleasure from fewer meals when you slow down to enjoy them. You'll also be more satisfied. What really is the difference between eating 10 cookies (or even the whole box) compared to eating just one in one sitting? You can express your joy with that one instead of scarfing down the 10 that you barely taste, and which can only put on pounds. You can increase the joy you get from one cookie if you eat more slowly. This also gives your stomach time to tell your brain that you are full and satisfied. You can consciously lengthen your perception of time to get more out of eating. Make the "cookie" a healthy activity and a healthy food.

Feel good about your small triumphs as you change. You may not go from ten to one cookie overnight, so give yourself a chance as you whittle away at the number you eat. Always feel optimistic, keep a sense of humor about yourself. Good times, good thoughts and a sense of humor will tend to eliminate negativity and stress. Progress is about having a one-year goal that you commit to, even going from ten cookies a sitting to one. You will probably move forward three steps and then go one step back as you improve--but you will improve. As the days go on and you make those small-step efforts for change, harmful food habits will occur less and less frequently. After you have eaten something you didn't need, consider how you felt before and after. What difference did it really make in your life? You just added weight to your body and for what?

What does contemplation give you? You can create your own plan of life given what you think. Thoughts go on forever and continuously.

You can stop them, improve them and totally change the way you exist--but only after you take the time to consider, contemplate and correct the beliefs you already have. **You will lose physical weight after losing any burdensome mental and emotional weight that influences why you overeat.** This concept is critical because it reveals why and how you became overweight and how to regain a healthy body weight for a better life. They are inseparable. This method is about permanence.

The *Inside-Outside Diet* is not about losing the very fundamentals that make you "you." Rather, it is about eliminating the thoughts that hold you back while having you understand how they influence your daily choices and how you function. You are not your thoughts, they are however what makes you move from point A to point B when you decide to make them important – and this can be changed.

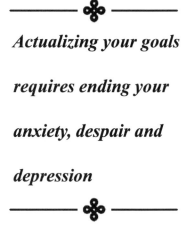

Actualizing your goals requires ending your anxiety, despair and depression

My goal for you is to gain greater clarity and understanding of what you do and why you do it. This can only be made more difficult when your attention span and memory are adversely affected by mood and mind-altering foods, additives and drugs. It is harder to change when cravings or addictions to food, drugs, alcohol or other substances either distract you or run your life. Even sleep deprivation or poor sleeping habits can bring out inner turmoil, and get you to turn to sugary foods or caffeine to keep you going. Fatigue is not useful in successfully probing your issues.

Your Past Thoughts

Whatever your age, the process of how you became overweight has been an ongoing occurrence with key moments of change in your life experiences. Those conscious and unconscious responses to living are formulated and, unless you make the effort to change them, remain obstinately the same. Inner decisions occur in an instant, while their emotional and physical repercussions evolve in a longer sustained time. **If you can make the connection between your inner and outer you, you will succeed.**

In holistic medicine, all mental, emotional and physical alterations must be present at the same time. Healing of the mental consciousness, though, takes precedence. It is more a determinant of the body, rather than the other way around, and allows for way more permanent change. Change the mind and you change your body.

Clients always ask me how to gain control over their thoughts so that they can pursue self discovery. Of the many preceding techniques, try this:

*To experience control over your thoughts, sit down when you're least distracted and observe the many thoughts that come to your mind --your thought production computer. You may recall a rare compliment from your boss or wish your mother would not always call with advice about your weight. Thoughts can come to you in words or pictures. Write all of them down as an exercise, but don't make the list of thoughts in words or pictures become your new mind's pursuit. Just watch them float by like balloons or clouds in the sky with your descriptions of what they are on them. If you feel as if your thoughts are running amuck (that is, they're coming at you fast and hard and you can't keep up), don't worry about writing them down. Rather, see how many appear to you and how endless they are. If you can't remember them all at this time, they will certainly come back again in slightly different forms. **The lesson from this exercise is to learn that you do not have to act on every thought and impulse – you can choose.**

*Habits change when they are replaced in your short term memory by new, different responses to old stimuli. Feeling anxiety?

You go for an apple or a healthy food until you resolve the basis of your anxiety and eliminate it. You can start to insert new thoughts into your mind and tell the stressful thoughts to stop. Remember that your old reactions took you down wrong paths and helped add on the weight. Ask yourself what was good about that thinking and how it helped you? How much good can you really attribute to guiding thoughts that took you down wrong paths?

Instead, you will build strength through repetition of healthier thoughts and actions. In time, you will develop better thoughts, better emotions, better ways of ridding negative or uncomfortable emotions when they arise. In this way, you use your mind to re-form your body and empower your life.

Often, good thoughts and bad thoughts are simultaneously in play. Good thoughts need to be amplified to counter and downplay negative thoughts. Even better is to satisfy your thoughts enough so that you can exist in a truly aware state where you do not even think at all. For too many thoughts, try this exercise to calm your mind.

The Thought-Extinguishing Exercise

This night-time exercise, for one, is good for releasing stressful obligations, helping you sleep better and resetting your mental power. It is good for mental emptying and releasing mental control.

You can do this exercise during the day if you feel yourself going into mental overload, but for the most part it's designed to do at bedtime to help you enjoy better health and a good night's sleep.

Start by making yourself comfortable, either lying down or sitting. Take a few deep breaths and let your muscles relax. Imagine a warm and comforting campfire in front of you and stare into the flames. Place whatever thoughts come to you into the fire. You can imagine them as having shape and form if you wish. One by one, look at each thought and then see it burn away in the fire, going up in smoke. This will take anywhere from five to 20 minutes, depending on how many thoughts come into your mind.

If imagining the fire is a problem for you, you might feel more comfortable picturing yourself standing by a river and letting your thoughts wash downstream. Or, you could stand on a mountain top and let your thoughts be blown away with the wind. Whatever image allows you to release your thoughts so that you feel relaxed and peaceful is fine.

If any particular thought offers resistance and keeps coming back to you, tell yourself that you don't have to deal with it right then--you can be reminded of it in the morning. Take a deep breath and let it out, mentally affirming that all situations eventually work themselves out. This might help you let go of a particularly difficult thought. In the world of thought, what makes an imagined outcome turn into a problem is believing that it will happen. Why do that? Let it be. Your mind must empty at night in order to heal.

Eight Concepts to Change

There are eight basic concepts to consider in contemplation when excess weight, overeating and lack of exercise describe you. Each one of these points is an important one to contemplate. You will probably have additional personal issues, but start here:

*Change your concept of work from its being negative to being useful. Thoughts that help you do this are changing your beliefs wherein the concept that work is about accomplishment, that work is enjoyable, that it stretches your skills and talents, and that it makes you social, feel happy and purposeful. Examine the whys and benefits of "work" as it relates to being physically active and exercising.

*Change your concept of "having time." Do you always feel rushed? That there's never "enough time," even though you know you often procrastinate or veg out in front of the TV and believe you deserve "the time off." The concept of having time is crucial to everyone's life. A relaxed, long-term approach to life is important or you will not put in the time to enjoy exercising, or not exercise with effort, not exercise regularly and, most counterproductive, think of all kinds of reasons not to work out at all. Everyone needs to slow down enough to have time to go peacefully through the day. How do you see your ability to slow down and take time to enjoy life?

   *Patience is a very important trait for you to contemplate. Impatience converts thoughtful purposeful responses into impulse reactions, prompts incorrect assumptions about what others did or didn't mean and makes you short-tempered when things don't go smoothly. When impatience becomes set into the foundation of your personality, failure follows. Patience is tied to a better way to deal with stress and time constraints.

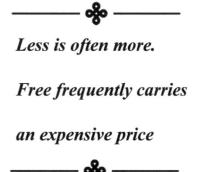

Less is often more.

Free frequently carries

an expensive price

   *Less is more. This is a concept that everyone who is overweight needs to implant in their mind. "More" is almost universally conceptualized in America as better, but it isn't. Remove the thought from internal concepts that you don't have enough. Instead think abundance. Think the world will provide what you need when it is necessary. Changing some of your views on worldly concepts is crucial to weight loss. You need to know what is and isn't really healthy and eliminate the faulty concepts you hold onto that are not true.

   *Understand the concept of hunger. If any practice can change your idea of hunger requiring instant gratification, it's a long fast. Long fasts can help you actually shift the concept of hunger from need and desperation to nothingness. Yes, it's true. You can minimize the significance of hunger for you to its being insignificant, *and with time and practice,* where hunger doesn't even exist.

Your concept of hunger is very important especially when you indulge your animalistic concept of eating and food. Do you eat like an animal? Barely chew and eagerly swallow without really tasting the food? Do you shovel food down and don't know when to stop? If you make hunger a matter-of-fact, non-primal drive, you can make other aspects of your life more important. This is very good and useful to do.

*Know how to increase your energy levels and comfort zones. Increasing your mental and emotional energy without wasting it on eating more food is a psychological technique that you can practice. A higher level of energy that you learn to direct away from food, helps keep you from putting your energy into physical eating. When you master this very real trait, you're getting closer to improvement, happiness and the best of your health.

*Financial survival. Don't let that feeling of deprivation carry over to this aspect of your life. You have to believe that you have enough, and that everything will turn out alright. Be sure that you will survive, financially and otherwise. Slow down, relax, enjoy life with what you have and be optimistic about the future. Feel faith.

*Think body concept. You must see your body as healthy, capable, and fit. You must enjoy your body!

In my opinion, all ailments are cured from the Inside to the Outside. Today's medicine has been focused on healing from the Outside inward. It is my belief that if you use all means available to you to improve your life--and use both Outside and Inside factors that help but don't hurt you-- you can finally resolve your original conflict and cure yourself.

You can actually get excited about losing weight. Make it for the time being, an enthusiastic drive in itself. The insights you gain from the inward pursuit of your drives, beliefs and emotions, all lead to greater self-knowledge and can be quite stimulating. Make weight loss a power-driven goal that you set.

When you encounter an outside obstacle, STOP, just don't pass over it. Stop and identify clearly what *inner* obstacle is at play. **Clearing up the clutter of your mind by removing any non-useful beliefs will result in increased willpower.**

Your Inner Life

You must have joy. You must have pleasure. You must be able to dump inner and outer tension when it arises, or at least, before you go to bed. You must be able to go to sleep peacefully without worries and tension.

It is all summed up with this principle that I want to emphasize again: *What thoughts you run in your mind will be the root key to your success.* What you think gives you freedom or not, compounds or builds tension or not, manifests your deeper self-esteem or breaks you down, shapes your beliefs in success, failure, pleasure and pain. It also motivates you to plan your future built on your most profound needs. **What matters is that you understand that every event in life does not have the same importance**. Traffic jams, for example, are annoying and no fun, but don't give them such emotional weight that you must eat to calm down. Learn to laugh, because there will always be obstacles in life and from within your self. Laughing and an inward sense of humor naturally correct your energy to an appropriate comfortable level.

If you set these priorities right and allow your tension to be released, your pleasure increases, your body changes to manifest your will and it will reflect your happiness. This is happiness that comes not from eating but rather, from a generous full expression of yourself. You will be busy doing the things you like and not have to snack and overeat. When you're really happy or doing what you should be doing in life, you won't have the drives to overeat--playing children rarely think about food. Other activities are much more joyous.

Of course, food will always be there for you to enjoy, but with emotional and mental balance, food will not be driving you. At this point, food will be in harmony with your needs and will not cause you harm. Food will no longer be an old automatic habit that you use to defuse tension or gain pleasure with calories. Food should be a small part of your life, a small health-giving necessity that you take time to prepare and consume. Your life will be full and you'll know true freedom.

The Search for Deliverance

You'll need to take time every day or week to work on yourself to understand why you do what you do. Getting to an understanding can be easy or difficult depending upon what drives, emotions and mind patterns you already have in place. Change occurs in an instant but you have to *make* the decision to change. Will and conviction, combined with the appropriate understanding, moves life inertia and bolsters your persistence to find the success you want.

For this quest, think about your weaknesses or self-defeating drives. What comes immediately to mind? *Write them down.* Then divide your life into three categories: the continuing emotions that you feel during the day, the persistent thoughts that get repeated over and over in your head, and your actualized drives--what you are working to accomplish every day.

Examine your emotions as they occur during the day, and you may quickly recognize that you're mostly sad, depressed, happy, worried or carefree during the day. Whenever you have an overriding emotional state and it affects your life in many ways, you have hit upon a major issue to examine and find out, within you, where it began. Here, you can start to work on the goal of turning your desire to be different, either for health, weight, happiness or success into reality. If you don't have one overriding obvious emotional state that sticks out as self-defeating, then go on to consider what other drives envelope your life.

Some drives may be obvious, like the compulsion to keep making money, but *why* do you want more money? Is it a symbol of something that means security or something that will build a protective wall around you to keep you from dying? Is having a lot of money your subconscious approach to never be out of control again, or is it to buy as many pleasurable things as possible? Are you working for rent only? Keep asking yourself questions. You might have a wrong foundation.

Extend this questioning from the moment you wake up, and ask yourself, why you eat a sugar filled breakfast, or a breakfast that adds on calories. Why do you call a particular friend when you need company, comfort or to have a good time? Is this friend also someone with overeating issues? Do any special activities in your lifestyle involve eating, or socializing with food as the backdrop? Your answers may open a can of worms that needs to be emptied, but it will also reveal how you developed up to this point. Being truthful and courageous will help remove any non-useful drives. **Clearing non-useful drives increases your conviction.**

You may discover that much of what you do is out of fear or as a means of survival without many emotional benefits. Are you living to keep from dying or living to live? You may see that much of what you do is about making sacrifices in one way or another for others. You may decide to alter your life based upon what drives are revealed from your self-evaluation. If you take time to examine how you function, you will retrieve the answers to your questions about yourself from your subconscious and see *why* you do what you do. Be honest with your answers—as this man in the following description has done.

I had a patient come to me with another typical situation, or drive, which I call a "run-on life," where the person is so busy that they never stop to consider what they are doing. In many cases, the patient is overweight and has some chest pain that may or may not end up being related to heart problems. Just getting such activity-addicted people to stop for even a moment to look at their lives can often be a monumental task. They tend to be much happier never looking at what is going on in their lives--until that moment hits when a fear of dying gets them to see a doctor.

Many people never look at their lives and proceed like a train that is about to derail and become something worse, a train wreck. So it was with my patient who I'll call Bob. What happened was that Bob made sure to keep his mind so busy that he had no time to deal with any serious issues about his health. He was adept at dealing with other serious issues like his work and job but as far as his health and his weight, he had no idea--or any information--about taking care of himself. Even when he came to see me, it took him three more months to make an effort and do something for himself.

There are a lot of smart people like Bob who just never take time to concern themselves with their own health. Fortunately for him, he had a personal revelation about his granddaughters and his not being there to participate in their future. This motivated him to see himself as someone responsible for his own well-being and theirs.

What Bob could do was follow the suggestions for eating healthier foods and taking supplements initially prescribed, but he was slow to do the real work--looking *Inside* for the real solutions. Typically American, Bob was good at doing the physical things but perplexed at working on invisible things, things he couldn't grasp with his hands. This meant he could put off probing his emotional and mental functioning. He had a typical Western attitude about health wherein he had never learned the importance of, or even existence of, his spiritual, emotional and mental well-being. Fortunately for Bob, grace and luck prevented him from catastrophe until he started making deeper corrections to his choices in life.

Creating Change

So, as with Bob, you may "think" on the surface that you want to lose weight, but in reality, you make almost no changes to drop the weight. Why? The truth, as this story shows, is that you don't take any action to accomplish what you "think" you are doing. When you accept this about your behavior, it is the first key to change. Figure out a realistic analysis of what you do. Doing and making strides, no matter how small, is greater strength than only thinking about it. But first:

Change the bad food to the good foods as I have listed, but also learn why you are living out such a harmful and un-fulfilling relationship with food. Your answers are important because it will reveal the underlying reasons for deceiving yourself and following harmful patterns that have been compelling you to make bad decisions and take bad actions. Sure, you can change what you eat and be better off, but change *why* you act, then eating better food becomes deeper and permanent. That principle will benefit you in many more ways your entire life.

Every small triumph is a gain for your eventual total triumph

Some clients tell me that when they discover the truths about what food does to them, they feel some despair! Don't dwell on the immediate reaction. Feeling that much despair usually means you are overburdened with damaging esteem beliefs from other causes already. Have faith and know that you can change anything about yourself once you realize the truth of what you are really doing. The truth gives you room to grow and you can create new experiences that give you joy, that reinforce truly healthy choices and help establish positive goals for you. Being aware of your hidden nature supports your placing in action your highest and healthiest goals! Never deny the truth.

Writing down ideas, revelations, wants, questions and answers is a tool you can use to objectively look at how you subjectively live your life. Here's your chance to go deeper and take note of what you actually do with your time:

*Get a piece of paper and write down your daily activities that show you how your lifestyle shapes up. Do this for seven days and then look over your activities and see what was necessary or unnecessary. What satisfied most accurately your goals versus what countered or wasted time. Then one at a time, look at all the negative acts and behaviors and contemplate why you did them. This can motivate you. Many negative, superficial actions point to one underlying mis-guided drive that once discovered, you can change.

*Write down what gives you pleasure or things that you like. Then write down what you dislike. Look over your lists to see what you are doing that harms you. This can help you more properly restructure higher goals. It doesn't mean that you should never experience a low, or experience frustration or even do something unpleasant, but you must have understanding of yourself to minimize the lows and direct yourself to the positive light.

*Make a separate list of what you do that is selfless and what is selfish. It is the balance of choices that must be corrected and not necessarily the total elimination of selfish traits. As long as you have a physical self, you need to take responsibility for your personal mental, emotional and especially bodily needs.

*Make another list of what you do that supports survival needs. This list is practical for you not to lose control of the real world.

*Make another list of what you are doing about achieving your goals. You may find that you have no pleasurable goals or childhood dreams left over to pursue with any sort of enthusiasm. This is probably not good for you. Everyone has a special purpose and should be able to live out a dream and have a fulfilling life. Your dreams and goals might rightfully change or mature with time and this is okay. To have none may indicate you need to refigure your life and contemplate what you are really doing. Seeing this list can help you organize your time and eliminate wasteful events and interactions. Also, don't discount people in your life, since you never exist alone.

I believe life is healthiest and weight automatically corrects itself best when people are functioning happily, joyously and with enthusiasm from the Inside to the Outside. If your life doesn't have any joy, change what you're doing or change your perception of what you're doing from negative to positive. **The only thing that matters in terms of emotional and psychological growth is knowing that it is not the event, the circumstance or the amount of food in front of you—it is about how you respond to it all!**

Know that work is necessary for survival. People will not always appear to make things happen for you, present you with a high-paying job or make life easier just because you wish it. Even a thousand years ago, people worked within their environment and did what they had to do to survive, whether it was planting a garden or raising livestock. We all work for what's necessary for survival, but in recent years, work has taken on the added dimension of satisfaction. If work doesn't offer contentment for you, think about how you can make it so. On the other hand, if you discover that you are overworking yourself, feel resentful or are simply doing a job that you are good at but hate, make plans to change.

*Some of your decisions will be big and some will be small. Any change that makes you more responsible for your joy will cut down on tension eating, depressive thoughts and the negative attitudes that stagnate within you to cause illness in your life.

*Another area of concern is how you think about yourself. Do you only think of yourself? Are you primarily concerned with not failing or block your progress by assuming your destiny is a lack of happiness? The ideal state is having a generally well-rounded opinion of your thoughts, emotions and drives. When any of these areas are out of balance or when they all have a predominantly negative theme, you've hit upon a key to the setbacks in your health, weight control and eventual freeing of life.

This self-analysis may seem difficult, but who else will really know the innermost parts of you, other than you. Who else can know your thoughts, emotions and drives better than you, the source itself? Have faith, and trust in yourself as you allow yourself to begin to expand your awareness from within, bit by bit. All the answers are there.

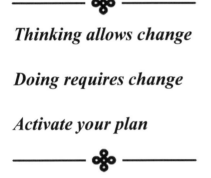

Thinking allows change

Doing requires change

Activate your plan

Remember the primary role of your mental and emotional functioning in your life style. Anything that promotes peacefulness will lessen the need to eat food. Only working non-stressful jobs will lessen the build-up of inner tension which often stimulates release through eating excess food. Discharging tension, stress or excess energy through physical activity will improve your health and curtail your use of food as a tension reliever. See the circumstances of your day optimistically and enthusiastically and you will have less stress.

Being positive can only be beneficial. If you force yourself to change your diet and feel deprived or cheated or believe you are "too weak" to do it, or if you perceive any forward motion to change as negative or "work," you'll rebound later and stop making the effort to change. I hope that this information will help convert you from negative to positive thinking so you understand why a positive outlook may be the first important step in becoming healthy. If you are negative, ask yourself how this belief is serving your conviction? It's limiting it.

Motivation is related to willpower but not the same. You can affect willpower with food, supplements and inner work, but motivation is something you originate totally within you. Start to get motivation by creating and inventing a life! Throw away false drives. What do you see yourself doing? How do you see yourself looking? These set images and goals in your deepest mind that may stimulate you. Be happy first! Be tolerant first. Be diligent, make plans and be persistent. All of this helps motivation.

The *Inside-Outside Diet* goes far beyond the weakness and imitation of dieting. This book includes practical techniques and solutions to change your Outside and your Inside, both of which are essential for losing weight, maintaining the weight you want and overall health for peace of body and mind.

There is a simpler you, basic, more creative nature, loving and just wanting to be loved and involved in the world of everything around you. You can still participate in life and achieve; follow your bliss, follow through and give yourself reasonable time to accomplish what you will.

To have pleasure, you need pleasure

To have joy, you need the absence of stress

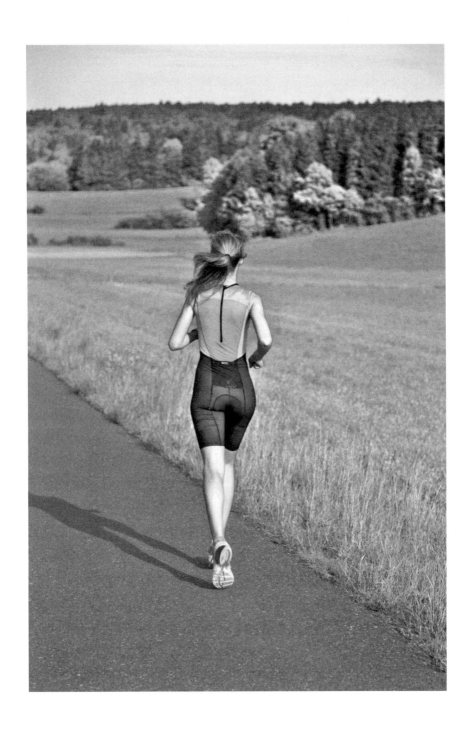

Part III:

Outside-In Changes for Weight Loss

Chapter Six

Food and Body Effects on your Health

I want to guide you through the holistic Outside information you need to know and implement to further enhance your knowledge of what a healthy weight really means. Outside-In healing involves anything you do to your body, and that includes 1) the food you choose, 2) the supplements taken and 3) the exercise you do regularly. These stabilize your body and place it in a better position to regain a healthy weight.

Use the external "outside-in" approaches to improve your body functions first, because they are easiest to accomplish and require the least willpower to do. The outside-in changes I'll suggest for you in terms of food and supplements--will increase your stamina, clarity and willpower. These changes from the outside and its effects on your body, give strength and support to your internal life and emotions (energy) and your inward thought processes (consciousness).

Even small improvements in food selection, supplements and lifestyle, increase your inner conscious powers that you will use to change on the inside. Each positive change brings you that much closer to your goal. Your physical body and emotional body will become in balance.

In 2006, I traveled to India to a Tibetan Bon refugee village and orphanage. I went there to determine the nutritional status and needs of the children and monks. What I saw there was an interesting comparison to American culture. While in the United States there is a lot of education lacking about the power of thoughts and emotions, there are still many people who have some healthy food knowledge and are making decisions to eat naturally.

In the Tibetan culture there is, by comparison, a very high cultural knowledge of the importance of your thoughts. However, these Tibetans are no longer living where their ancestors grew up and do not have the same food. Neither has their culture developed an education about the effect of foods on the body--unlike what's currently available in the West. Unnatural foods never existed in the Tibetan culture and have never become a part of their teachings for health. So now that soda pop and processed foods have entered the Tibetan's food lists, they are starting to have hypertension, diabetes and the beginnings of overweight issues. With the deterioration of the body, they will start to have a loss of ability to focus, clarity and evenness of mood--exactly opposite to the manner of disease progression in the United States in some ways. Your body, emotions and mind are all connected and affect each other *Inside to Outside* and *Outside to Inside*. Food, exercise and supplements are important for regaining inward health.

Your physical body is not only important, but crucial to understand because you experience life through it. Things you do to your body may not be as lasting as what you change about your emotions and thought, but physical changes are the easiest to correct. Lifelong permanent good physical health occurs when you make all the correct inner mental, emotional and physical adjustments. Your body is a physical temple that houses the real you whose nature is creative, happiness and peace. So let's create that peace and support inside and out.

Standard medical texts, and even nutritional texts, will leave out much of what you need to know about food, health and nutrition. And, there's no argument that the food you take into your body has an effect on you, besides sating hunger. Foods can have drug-like effects on your body, a condition like addiction you want to avoid normally.

You can start the weight-loss process by making adjustments, little by little, in your food choices. Cut the sugar. Limit the fats and choose the natural ones. Start to include physical improvements like exercise and make a commitment to a lifestyle change that will improve your inner mental and emotional attitudes. Your mental clarity, persistence, evenness of mood, decreased anxiety and increased willpower can all be improved through exercise or just moving your body. These helpful improvements set the stage for you to at last, discover and alter your beliefs and emotional patterns that originally underlie your overeating compulsions.

Identifying hunger

True hunger is a bodily sensation you feel in your abdomen signaling you to eat. It's an urge to consume something. Any deficiency of nutrients such as minerals, vitamins, amino acids, essential fatty acids or even water can cause abnormal eating drives. The need for these nutrients makes you consume food in an attempt to provide what your body may be requiring.

Here are a number of points for you to remember:

*Know the difference between **thirst versus hunger.** Realize that it is easy to physically mistake thirst for hunger and eat unnecessarily. Take a moment to consider what you're really feeling when you think you're feeling hungry. Discern whether or not you may be dehydrated and then, even so, drink a large glass of mineralized water before eating. This may satisfy that "hunger" and prevent another episode of confused eating. As you take in fewer calories than before, you will lose weight and inherently feel better with proper hydration.

*Recognize your **need for electrolytes.** You cannot sweat or urinate without losing salts from your body. If you feel a specific drive for something salty, you know you are in need of those electrolytes. Instead of wandering aimlessly to the food pantry and eating anything, intentionally take some magnesium or add low sodium salt to your next meal. While salt has been downplayed as a bad thing that can cause high blood pressure, it is actually the sodium in it that's responsible. Magnesium can lower blood pressure and be better for your heart. And remember: the more you exercise and perspire, the more you need salt replacement. Most bottled waters sold today are actually distilled tap water that contain no minerals. Drinking this kind of water will deplete your minerals, make you feel nauseated or weak and drive false "hunger."

It is okay to use sea salt or low sodium salt in your food preparation and occasionally supplement with magnesium. Many patients of mine in the dry climate of Arizona describe needing salts. Often this translates for some to feeling the need to eat salty chips, especially on long drives in the car where boredom can also set in. Supplementing magnesium and other salts can prevent this unnecessary calorie consumption.

*Know that **any essential nutrient you're deficient in can stimulate body-based drives to eat.** With this in mind, I always recommend that people take supplements from a high-quality supplement manufacturer. The primary nutrients you need to take are vitamins, co-factors and minerals including trace minerals. Also take essential fatty acids such as fish oil or flaxseed oils. Since the body requires 30 to 75 grams of amino acids a day, be sure to get all the essential aminos in your food. I take a high-quality basic nutrient and mineral supplement, essential omega 3 and omega 6 fatty acids, and occasionally I supplement with trace minerals on an empty stomach, which increases their absorption. I'm also sure to get amino acids from my food such as egg whites, nuts and seeds, lean meat, or legumes and lentils that complement each other nutritionally.

Sugar, salt and fats seem to be genetically hard-wired in the body to create driving sensations of pleasure, security and well-being, even though these nutrients cause damage when in excess. Be aware that poor restaurants often overdue these ingredients to your detriment, all in an attempt to make you return for more food and business. Excessive use of these ingredients, particularly from restaurants, also lead to overeating and too many calories.

To be different

You have to *BE* different

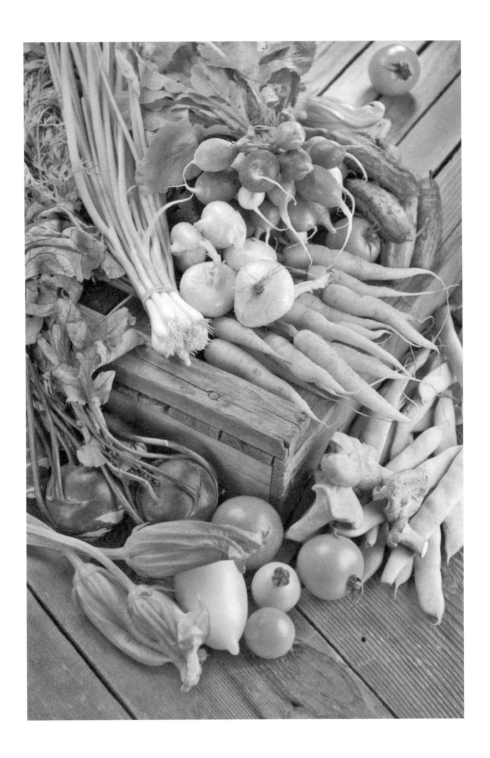

Chapter Seven

The Benefits of
Holistic Nutrition and Lifestyle

What do you really need to know about food and nutrition?

Simply, the food you eat, and when and how you eat it can either make you healthy or sick. Too much food, or the wrong food for your individual body constitution can make you ill and overweight. Missing nutritional elements, due to nutrient-deficient food can lead to cellular and organ starvation. Unnatural toxic elements from manufacturing or a toxic environment can cause ill health, too. What this tells you is that food is important to your health and survival in many ways.

Unfortunately, most people do not regard food as having much effect on their health. Potato chips or pork rinds, they think, are basically food products, therefore, these high-fat and processed foods are okay to eat as any foods. Not so. Eating is one thing you do every day for your entire life. Like the air that you breathe (often affected by smoking or pollution) and the water that you drink (often including the additives fluoride, arsenic, polychloral biphenyls, nitrates and heavy metals) these environmental influences and the food you consume are the constant life activities that expose your body to health or illness.

When it comes to food quality, I have two main concerns. There can be essential nutrients missing from the food due to over-production or processing losses, and there can be unnatural compounds in the food that can act like poisons in your body--compounds like mercury in fish, especially tuna. There is also a third element in food that cannot quite be measured and it's called "life energy." This refers to that invisible element of what food is meant to impart to us--sustenance and energy--but which can be disturbed or missing when food is produced from a caged, abused or sick animal versus the healthier life of a wild, well-treated animal. I consider all three aspects of food (nutrients, toxins and life energy) important.

From this, lesson one would be: Do not underestimate the powerful health or unhealthy effects of the food you eat. Many clients who have been on a healthier diet and those who have not have something in common: a youth spent eating too much junk food. Twenty years of youth is a long time and you can actually become contaminated, nutrient depleted and ill early in life from your earlier food decisions.

Unfortunately, some of our contemporary foods don't nourish any of the body at all, they only fill it. Grocery stores and even health food stores carry foods that are damaging to your health. With these foods we take in petroleum products, heavy metals, pesticides, herbicides, insecticides and a few other assorted pollutants. To avoid eating poisons from the very shelves of your grocery store, you need to gain some education about what foods are healthy for you and which foods can cause illness.

You're not alone if you feel you're missing essential knowledge about nutrition, food and your health. They are subjects that tend to be missing from our educational system. You will have to gain this education for yourself. It's the only way to be properly in control of your life and health. Food companies will usually only tell you what is best about their products so you buy them. Doctors are also mostly undereducated in nutrition so they can't advise you today either.

What's best for you? Holistic nutrition.

Holistic nutrition refers to foods that nourish the whole body and spirit. Eating holistically, and finding helpful foods that lead to proper balance and function, has become a real challenge in today's market place.

In general, people watching their weight tend not to look at nutrition holistically. Traditionally, they always focus on sugar content, fat content, carbohydrate content and "counting calories." Dieticians may focus more on classifying food in terms of carbohydrate, protein, and saturated fat, using terms like "the glycemic index." Useful information, but good long-term health calls for considering vitamin, mineral, trace mineral and essential fatty acid content. Also, you can consider alkaline/acid and ayurvedic food properties. Even greater benefits can come from discovering which foods really work for you as an individual.

The foundation of holistic nutrition is eating naturally-grown foods in season, prepared in natural ways, in good combinations. Other considerations include differences between eating raw versus cooked food with natural fire or in a stove versus using a microwave. Raw food for example, still retains its natural enzymes valuable for digestion. Finding good, minimally-processed foods in stores, however, has become difficult. Eating what should be a natural diet has become almost impossible for the majority of people. This is mainly because of unnatural food additives and the similar use of natural compounds from unnatural foods like canola oil, (thought to be a bonus for low-fat, non-stick cooking!) cottonseed oil or palm kernel oil.

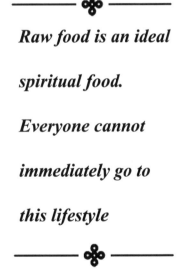

Raw food is an ideal spiritual food. Everyone cannot immediately go to this lifestyle

If you're lucky enough to have a patch of land, the best food might be what you plant and care for in your own garden, composting your organic wastes into your soil, watering with filtered or quality well water. Food raised in this way will also have your personal care and love in it. This adds a "life energy" factor to your food. You can pick it ripe and eat it fresh, getting the fullest nutritional and energy value. Many foods offer the best energy and nutrition when you eat them uncooked or only lightly cooked. Foods have a life and a vibration to them that is just as real as your thoughts and emotions.

Eating raw foods tends to maintain the best of this life force. For example, you can replant a fresh healthy carrot, and it will have enough life force to continue growing. But this life energy is often degraded or missing because of modern day farming practices and food processing. Although the chemical content may test out the same, a fresh vegetable obviously has something that its canned counterpart does not. Freezing, although a superior method of long term food storage, also takes the life away from foods. Overcooking foods or exciting their molecules in a microwave can also debilitate the final food quality and consequently our health.

Heating, that is, cooking, often changes the actual chemicals in the food for the worse. Look at all the oily French fries Americans eat, even though research shows that heating oil over 280-360 degrees causes carcinogenic changes in the oil. Growing your own food or eating a large amount of food uncooked may sound unrealistic now, but change is a step by step process. As you change your dietary habits for the better, you get closer to another change that seemed impossible from where you were before. Just having a good food perspective and recipe book can be instrumental in change to healthier food.

Farming with vast quantities of synthetic chemicals to get higher yields with less weeds and bugs has contaminated everything we eat. Our foods and water end up containing pesticides, herbicides (like atrazine), insecticides and even some heavy metals, all of which are neurotoxic to our bodies. Our brain and central nervous system, as well as our peripheral body nerves, contain high amounts of fatty acids. When agricultural chemicals along with abnormally long-chain fatty acids infiltrate and become infused in these nerve cells, they dysfunction. Unfortunately, if these specialized nerve cells die, they usually cannot be replaced. Contaminated nerves can short-circuit.

These unnatural chemicals can also cause infertility, birth defects and a host of other problems including cancer and chronic fatigue. If you eat organic food, it is still possible that it was grown in ground that was previously chemically treated, and some traces of contamination may still exist.

Even if the soil does not contain these agricultural pollutants, it might be the 40th crop on that land in 10 years. And without allowing the land to lie fallow and then rotating contrasting crops to replenish the soil, the crops produced will lack the trace minerals that would make it truly healthy. Overproducing crops is not new. The Old Testament instructs people not to plant their land every year, ancient sage advice that remains true.

Stock only healthy fruits and vegetables in your home

Despite the farmer's best intentions, the land may not escape the consequences of modern farming. My parents have farmed in Iowa their entire lives and tell me that even on some isolated smaller farms you cannot drink the well water because of large amounts of nitrates contaminating the underlying aquifer. Environmental pollution has extended itself to all areas of the world where once pristine nature thrived. The history of scientific manipulation without long term sustainable studies has damaged our earth and health.

I mentioned earlier that 20 years of youth probably exposed you to some measure of food not meant for human consumption. Recent studies further indicate that if you are over the age of 20, you almost certainly carry a burden of heavy metal or neurotoxic chemicals in your body that at some level, I believe can cause overt illness. Current science does not give much thought to low level contaminants, and it is difficult to link them to health problems in people. However, I believe that if something definitively is toxic at a certain level then it must still have ill effects on people below the test level range. An example of this is canola oil touted as a healthy oil when it still contains 1 percent of a toxin called euric acid. What's more, it seems like simple math, that ingestion of low levels over time will eventually amount to high levels. I recommend you test the water anywhere you plan to live. No matter how pristine the land looks, who knows what mining or manufacturing plant was in the neighborhood 60 years ago or what the ground water contains.

Although it costs a little more, eat organic foods when you can. For one thing, by eating organic, you cast a vote for moving our society away from agricultural chemicals. Even if some "organic" products are not quite as pure as the label says, in the long run, you will allow less harmful chemicals to enter your body. "Organic" meats cost significantly more, but because animals are higher up the food chain, non-organic meats could have much higher levels of hormones and other contamination than non-organic meats.

If you eat animal products at all, then it is best if the animals are raised in a natural, low-stress environment without chemical stimulants. Animals raised in the wild have a vibrant energy that caged animals lack. The same holistic application applies to fish "farmed" for restaurants and grocery stores. Do you think it natural for any fish to be farmed? Without any sense of a natural life, these fish live in overcrowded waters eating manufactured food along with their own feces. On top of that, many farmed salmon are given artificial coloring for a brighter red appearance.

Another recent study of farm-raised salmon showed the fish to contain 14 cancer-causing chemicals and advised eating it no more than once a month. But isn't that ridiculous, if you find out something is poisonous, would you recommend eating less of it? Of course not. You would say eat none of it! I never eat farm-raised fish. While fish should have been one of the best foods you could eat, it has become something that you should not eat because of its heavy metal and/or industrialized pollutant contents. Fish have also become over fished in nature.

Normally one of the best meats to eat, fish offers a very lean source of protein and therefore, amino acids; however, the problems have come to outweigh the benefits. Contamination with synthetic chemicals and heavy metals, most notably mercury, has become widespread in oceans, rivers and lakes. It is best to check your local internet report on what fish are considered edible for your area. You might be surprised to see what's in your local internet fish report.

Nearly all fish are contaminated with heavy metals

Experts particularly recommend avoiding shark, king mackerel, tuna, sea bass, marlin, halibut, pike, walleye, white croaker, largemouth bass, swordfish and Gulf of Mexico oysters. Fish from the Pacific Northwest, Scandinavia and Alaska are probably the least contaminated. Studies suggest that mercury causes neurological damage which may play a part in autism, ADD, ADHD, Parkinson's disease and Alzheimer's. The increasing numbers of adults and children diagnosed with these illnesses in the last 30 years raises great concerns about how abnormal food trends and contamination have affected our population.

Mercury in fish did not suddenly become a recent problem. The regulating bodies and the fish industries finally decided to *tell* us it's a problem. To an extent, we can blame ourselves for relying upon an industry which makes money off a product to inform us that it's dangerous. **Eight to ten percent of child bearing age women already**

have enough mercury in their bodies to cause motor, sensory and intelligence problems in their newborns. Still, the FDA recommends that women can still have half a can of albacore tuna per week providing they have no other seafood during that time. Knowing this, would you want any?

It has taken 30 years to break through the truth about the dangers of tobacco; and fish contamination, a giant environmental, consumer and food producer's catastrophe, appears to go back nearly as far. Unfortunately, a lot of body builders and dieters have grown accustomed to having those nice cans of tuna as a cheap and tasty source of protein. They are trading short term results and economics for a future of mercury contamination and heavy metal burden within their bodies.

From a holistic standpoint, we know there is more to food than how many calories it has or whether it is carbohydrate, protein or fat. Unfortunately western medicine has come to focus on little more than that. This may explain why our American health has sunk so low and obesity has become so high. Fat, protein and carbohydrates sustain life through energy burning calories. However, there are many other ingredients that go into making a healthy life.

Let's take them one at a time.

*Fats are vital to good health. They are most commonly found in animal meats, nuts, seeds, eggs and oils. Although nuts, eggs and animals are products or creatures of nature, they can be contaminated with synthetic compounds. Oils on the other hand, pose more of a modern problem. Some naturally derived oils like canola, cottonseed or even palm kernel are used by manufacturers in mass-produced products because they are so cheap. When you read the label on a product, you will find that these oils land in most chip or fried products. These oils come from plants not normally considered a source of food and, therefore, they have not been included within the digestive evolution of most human consumption. That alone should make these oils prime

suspects for many of our modern ailments and illnesses. I recommend using the more natural olive, sunflower or perhaps sesame oils. They are easily digestible and compatible for most people.

Abnormally long-chain fatty acids have been found in higher than average numbers in the cells and mitochondria of people diagnosed with ADD, ADHD, Parkinson's Disease, Alzheimer's Disease and other nerve tissue illnesses. These extra long-chain fatty acids have been described as brittle and deform cellular membranes. These abnormal fats are found in oils such as canola and cottonseed, along with the margarine and oleos that we have been consuming for the last 30 years in the quest to lose weight. Trans fats have only recently been identified as causing illness, yet they have been in the American industrialized diet for decades. This is an example of why you should not wait for science to test something unnatural before you stop using it. **If something is unnatural, and there are natural alternatives available, always go for the natural product.**

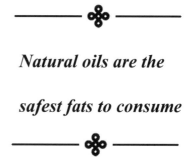

Natural oils are the safest fats to consume

Because some studies have associated high levels of cholesterol with cardiovascular illness, medical practitioners put a lot of value into checking your lipoprotein and cholesterol levels. In my practice, I could practically care less about cholesterol unless a patient has familial hypercholesterolemia with cholesterol levels approaching several hundred because these people consequently have a dramatically higher risk of heart disease. Pushing cholesterol levels below 170 has now been associated with an increased risk of stroke.

If you don't eat enough cholesterol your body will manufacture it, that's how important your evolutionary self put into cholesterol. Any substance that the body actually makes must have an important purpose. Cholesterol serves an important function in bile for fat digestion and actually comprises part of your cellular membranes. It is also used to make the important sex hormones in the body. What I recommend with heart and blood vessel disease concerns for cholesterol is eat more healthful food choices, particularly with less use of animal fats and dairy products from cows. When you get more vegetables into your diet, less fat, fewer carbohydrates and do a little exercise, the cholesterol will come down and take care of itself for most people. Fish oil or omega 3 essential fatty acids, taken at 3-6 grams a day may protect your vascular health, no matter what your triglyceride and cholesterol levels.

The use of liver-stressing synthetic medications, like the statin drugs, chemically lower cholesterol rather than bringing it into a natural, sustainable balance. This stresses and can actually damage the liver. Statin drugs dramatically lower one of the most important vitamin co-factors in your body, Coenzyme Q 10. Because statin drugs may lower blood urea nitrogen and creatinine levels, some people with borderline kidney functioning are now taking them, too. A natural food called red yeast rice was actually removed from the free market at one time by the FDA because it was too similar to a synthetic pharmaceutical product. Red yeast rice worked to reduce cholesterol, perhaps without side effects, so its removal from the market may actually say more about the FDA siding with industry.

*Nuts, animal meats, and eggs contain protein with *amino acids*. Usually people think of meat when they think of amino acids, but almost all foods contain a mixture of protein, carbohydrates, fiber and fat. Whether it is ultimately better to eat foods from the lower food chain will be debated for some time, so I suggest you eat according to your conscience and bodily needs. You can consider this a word of wisdom or a word to the wise.

If possible, find the source of protein that is most compatible with your body's evolution. I consider raw vegetarian eating to be the most healthy and spiritual form of living. Infants and children *must* have enough protein in their diet - or brain, other dysfunctions and even death can occur. I do not recommend vegetarian diets for children and infants unless they are highly monitored, given regularly nutritionally balanced food and are supplemented.

Some amino acids are considered "essential" because the body cannot make them, so we must consume them. Vegetarians in particular must be very careful to get all eight essential amino acids. Vegetarians must also be careful to get enough vitamin B12, zinc, calcium, iron and vitamin D. Many people fail to get all their eight essential amino acids because they rely on meat, and not all meats contain all the amino acids. Eggs are one of the few complete amino acid foods, providing all of the amino acids our bodies need. Quinoa is a grain that also contains all eight essential amino acids. Amino acids convert into muscle but they also become converted into polypeptides which function as neurotransmitters in our bodies.

The body has certain neurohormones and neurotransmitters such as serotonin and dopamine that are important in body communication and creating the feelings of peace or satiety. These neurochemicals are formed in the body from specific amino acids which if they are deficient could create a hormonal imbalance. Protein and amino acids can be consumed to balance these key bodily hormones and raise their levels to an appropriate level.

The following amino acid therapies relate to multiple neurohormonal products such as norepinephrine, dopamine and serotonin levels in your body. Neurohormonal imbalance affects many of our clinical symptoms of disease. I use amino acid neurohormonal therapy for a limited time for conditions such as depression, insomnia and cravings and then allow natural foods to develop stability.

*The neuro-transmitter serotonin is derived from L-tryptophan or 5-HTP and is found in turkey. The catecholamines like epinephrine come from the amino acid l-tyrosine. It is available in almost all meats except pork.

*GABA or gamma amino benzoic acid is a neurotransmitter derived from L-glycine, L-taurine and L-theanine. Endorphins are derived from d-phenylalanine, and the amino acid L-glutamine provides a fuel source for brain cells.

*Dopamine is derived from phenylalanine and is the "pleasure molecule" that satisfies restless behavior and overeating.

*Thyroid supplementation: I recommend almost everyone take supplemental iodine with the amino acid tyrosine for two months when people are overweight. I also add other thyroid nutrients to people's regimen when they are overweight. Iodine, thyroid nutrients and essential fatty acids will be necessary for you to have your body function optimally. Despite all this, you may still need thyroid hormone replacement if your body still responds inadequately.

The lack of these neuro-transmitters can contribute to depression, difficulty sleeping, lack of attention, anxiety, emotional instability, food cravings, substance abuse and addictions. That's why I regularly suggest trying a few weeks of specific amino acid replacement therapy before considering synthetic anti-depressants. Of course, I would also suggest cognitive emotional and belief system investigation at the same time. The psychological problems and underlying abnormalities will almost always precede the symptoms. The link between body, thought and emotions can be particularly easy to trace within this area of neurohormonal health.

If you have high blood pressure, take MAO inhibitors, take SSRI's, are manic depressive, get migraine headaches or have low blood pressure, see a medical doctor before supplementing with specific amino acids. Avoid inflammatory supplements and foods that provide GLA due to inflammation. Always see a holistic-minded doctor before trying to make physical changes to your life. Nutrients can have drug like effects on your body as can food itself.

<u>Natural Nutrients and Supplements for Weight Loss</u>

I recommend very few nutrients to be taken continually.

Get your body well stocked with all the essential vitamins, minerals, trace minerals, essential amino acids (particularly if you have food cravings), and essential fatty acids. Most people leave off the omega-6 fatty acids but current recommendations are that you need omega 6 fatty acids in a 1:4 ratio to omega 3 fatty acids. You will also want to pre-load your body with the natural anti-free radical protectors d-alpha mixed tocopherols and tocotrienes.

Natural *vitamin E* protects the cell and the cell membranes from rampant metabolic oxidation. These molecules are your natural protection from cancer. Your body can take in vitamin E and store it to some degree. Your body can also store all the other fat soluble vitamins such as vitamins A, D, and K. The water soluble vitamins such as vitamin C and the B vitamins need to be replaced daily.

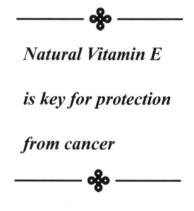

Natural Vitamin E

is key for protection

from cancer

Along with natural vitamin E you also need zinc, selenium and vitamin C to protect your body from oxidation. There are other anti-oxidant products advertised in the health-care markets such as grapeseed extract, but to me they are not as natural as mixed tocopherol vitamin E. When in doubt, choose the most natural effective products. On a cellular level where everything really happens, you are protected by vitamin E complexes, safeguarding your cellular life.

Chromium and vanadium are trace minerals important in glucose management. Omega 3 fatty acids protect the neurohormonal balance and counter the inflammation in your blood vessels. Fiber is in most fruit and vegetables, helps bowel motility and helpful synergistic bacteria located there.

Coenzyme Q10 is a necessary energy catalyst in your body. L-carnitine helps the body utilize fat in the cells. Alpha lipoic acid helps with glucose metabolism. Quercetin, at a dosage of 100mg a day can be helpful to regaining your best healthy body. You may want to use all these nutrients initially for two months in case you're deficient but I do not recommend you take them continually.

Because excess carbohydrates convert to fat, many people advocate the radical reduction of carbohydrate consumption; however, many of these higher-carb foods offer your best sources of nutrition: vegetables. With the global selection of vegetables available, your body may be incompatible with some of them. But they are also one of the most natural groups of foods within your evolutionary frame of reference. Most vegetables contain carbohydrates along with vitamins, minerals and enzymes. Enzymes come in broad varieties, performing numerous functions such as aiding in digestion and helping to cleanse toxins from our bodies. Probably the best and most universal class of food: vegetables contain good dietary fiber which helps the bowel eliminate wastes. Most vegetables also contain low amounts of calories. They are the ideal food in everyone's diet. I recommend eating all the nutrient dense, non-starchy vegetables you enjoy, along with fruits and an occasional meat if you so desire.

Another natural carbohydrate-bearing food, fruits are some of the most healing foods. A raw apple a day really may keep the doctor away. Regardless of what the diet doctors may have told you, eating fruits is not really a problem. Drinking fruit juices though, unnaturally magnifies the concentration and rate of sugar consumption. For this reason I do not recommend juice diets. So avoid drinking all juices, but eat fruits in season, nature's perfect food. They have a high water content like the human body and contain important vitamins like A, C, some B's and usually vitamin E (in the seeds). They also contain many basic and trace minerals.

Fruits are low in fat and high in the fiber necessary for effective working of your main elimination system, the colon. Fruits are low in calories as long as you don't overeat them or concentrate them in juices. Citrus foods, like oranges and lemons, however, are initially very acidic and some people can't tolerate them, so I recommend limiting your consumption of them. Choosing more alkaline fruits on the food intake scale will usually be better for your body.

What gives carbohydrates their bad name is their sugar content. Sugar is a real problem today! In the United States, sugar consumption has gone from 15 pounds per person a year to 175 pounds. This is a deadly amount of a substance that physiologically resembles illegal stimulants. Physically, sugar can lead to compromised immune systems, obesity, diabetes and other complex bodily problems. Emotionally, sugar has detrimental effects on your mood, personality, attention span and self-control, doubtlessly playing a part in much of today's personality and mood complaints. I recommend avoiding sugar altogether which still means you will get your 15 pounds per year just because so many foods that we eat "secretly" contain sugar.

Sugar tastes good so it sells the food off the grocery store shelves and brings customers back to the restaurants. Adding extra sugar, salt and animal fats to any food usually raise their taste levels. They also raise health risks. Be careful of this trick in the restaurants you visit. Some day all restaurants will list the sources of their food and water on the back of their menus.

Another problematic food is *cow dairy products*. While a natural product, some studies have linked cow dairy to diabetes, gastrointestinal problems and even poor cardiovascular health. Yes, it is often praised because it contains calcium, but so does cement. For women, good health calls for higher amounts of *calcium*, but often the call is not answered. You can get much more usable calcium in vegetables, such as in kale, broccoli and collard greens. There is also growing concern of whether milk contains hormones that have been fed to cows in the dairy industry. While some people can eat dairy without problems, many more people would be better off eating cheeses and yogurt made from goat's or sheep's milk. Apparently these animals have lived with mankind since an earlier time in our evolution because fewer people develop allergies to the dairy products made from their milk. If you are experiencing gastrointestinal problems, I suggest you eliminate cow dairy totally for 2 months to test yourself. If you are going to eat cow dairy products, I suggest you eat clarified butter (ghee), cultured yogurt or cottage cheese.

Many people are deficient in magnesium because it is easily lost in food processing. When you are deficient you may experience muscle aches and fatigue, high blood pressure and other symptoms. Trace minerals are minute quantities of minerals in the body that are essential for some bodily enzymatic processes. Examples are copper (necessary for elastin and melatonin production), vanadium (necessary for sugar metabolism) and chromium (necessary for sugar metabolism, i.e. diabetes). Trace minerals, such as molybdenum and boron are often overlooked in our supplements too, and they are important for good health. In laboratory studies, animals lacking trace minerals have had total system failure and even death.

Essential fatty acids that the body cannot manufacture on its own are probably the most overlooked dietary deficiency in our modern day eating habits. Easy symptoms to recognize are dry eyes, dry skin and brittle nails, but again the potential for calamity on a cellular level is much more significant. Fatty acids form the protective barriers around each of our cells and within our cell's energy producing mitochondria. To a greater extent, they also protect nerve and brain tissue. The potential for human disease from a lack of the correct essential fatty acids is enormous, particularly with our recent modern day practice of eating trans and hydrogenated oils and butter substitutes. The unnatural oils and spreads have the additional danger of containing vegetable oils comprised of abnormally long-chain fatty acids. Omega 3 fatty acids are also important for neurohormonal balance.

Addictions and Cravings

Addictions and cravings are body-based drives that give rise to certain emotions that those addictions and cravings make us believe we "need" something. These cravings require your being courageous and willing to look into the mental and emotional needs you're feeling when the craving occurs. It's healthier to generate positive emotions and feelings the natural way--by our thoughts, through non-harmful activities and by our willingness to live life more openly and receptively. You can have a natural high, without drugs or excess food. It achieves what should be everyone's goal of responsible consciousness.

What is it that you're really craving when you want a chocolate bar or a liter of soda pop or even a drug? What energy are you trying to reach, generate or distract? What do these substances really do to your sense of fulfillment, pleasure and conscious freedom? Could you imagine the feeling the addictive food gives you and consciously produce it without eating, drinking or ingesting them? The miracle is that the mind can produce any emotion, but it takes practice. You can allow any situation to envelope you by imagining it and then use mental exercises to build the presence of the emotion that you want.

You can have food cravings and addictions due to a relative lack of key neurotransmitters. Amino acid supplementation may give temporary assistance on the physical level to help alleviate certain addictions and cravings. To help you from the Outside-In, I recommend that you do a trial of balancing specific amino acids for the particular cravings that follow and see how they can help relieve them.

If you are dealing with a drug or food addiction I suggest you see a holistic doctor for an evaluation. Chromium, trace mineral and/or amino acid therapy can make the transition away from addiction easier. In some severe cases, alternative doctors may choose to use IV amino acid therapy. Psychological inquiry of original causes of your emotional problems will be imperative in dealing with addictions.

*A need for *sweets* can be treated by supplementing with chromium, vanadium, biotin and l-glutamine. *L-glutamine* is a fuel source for brain cells. Chromium and vanadium are necessary for correct glucose metabolism and are important for diabetics to supplement every so often.

*If you have the habit of consuming *liquid sugar drinks* such as soda pop or breakfast juices, the amount of sugar you have been taking in may be de-stabilizing your sugar balance and contributing to diabetes or metabolic syndrome. You must stop using all soda pop and quit consuming sugars to allow your body to even itself out from hyper and hypoglycemic episodes. Your body will feel the result of cutting out the sugar! For one week or so, you will probably feel worse but then the reversal happens. Your body should become steady in its glucose maintenance. Be aware that a need for sweets often ties into a need for emotional security.

*Chocoholics are often proud of their expertise on *chocolate*, and happily tell you about their addiction for the stuff. Designer chocolate may be the rage, but think again. It's not a health food, even though it's a plant. I consider chocolate an overused herb as it lowers energy levels and contains caffeine. Forty ounces of chocolate can kill a 16 pound dog. To wean yourself off chocolate, try this: Take supplements of *d-phenylalanine* or *GABA* (gamma amino benzoic acid) which are types of amino acids. And, examine when you feel the greatest need for chocolate and why it offers calmness and stress relief. Chocolate seems to lower or divert tension energy.

*A need for *heavy starchy meals* can be treated with *5-HTP* (5 hydroxy tryptophan) and GABA. If you have depressive elements to your life or difficulty sleeping, these psychological issues also must be addressed.

*A craving for *alcohol* can be treated with GABA and 5-HTP. Obviously, the need to probe the meaning of your alcohol intake is an inside evaluation of your lifestyle.

*A need for *stimulants, such as caffeine,* can be treated with *l-tyrosine* and high DHA fish oil. When you are overweight you need to eliminate coffee and other stimulants to finally get off the roller coaster ride they create. To be sure that your need for stimulants isn't body-based rather than an internal drive, see your medical doctor and have your thyroid functions checked out at some point.

Say no to stimulants, msg or heavy foods that alter your mood. Get used to natural life energy and flow. Initially, coming off emotional food may feel like a withdrawal, but in 1-2 weeks you will stabilize.

Herbal Approaches To Weight Loss

Because I believe it so important for permanent health and weight loss for you to correct the powerful inner causes of overeating, I do not believe in using herbs as a helpmate over the long term. If you insist that you need an herb to counter eating drives, then you are really not working on clarifying and then conquering your internal abnormal eating drives to begin with. Strong appetite suppressants or amphetamine-like herbs work against your ultimate inner control.

I do recommend the *occasional* use of herbs to intermittently balance your health. Herbs are not meant to be taken long term and may pose risks to health since they must be detoxified by the body like any other medication. Teas are the best type of herb for intermittent use.

The following herbs have been used for diabetes and/or weight control:

*Peppermint, can be used as a tea to satisfy hunger. It has been known to calm the stomach and has been used by many cultures over time and has safety of use on its side.

*Perfect Peace, is a blend that I use of Roman chamomile, German chamomile, nettles and tangerine peel (chen pi, a Chinese herb). All of these herbs have been used for a long time. This combination tends to balance all three ayurvedic doshas: kapha, weight gain; pitta, digestive ailments; vata, mental stimulation, stress and anxiety.

*Hoodia, a newly discovered herb from Africa, is believed to suppress hunger. Temporarily useful, it is not well tested, researched or comes with a bona fide history of use outside of Africa. It may be of value like other herbs for temporary assistance in weight loss by acting on appetite suppression. Eventually you have to do it on your own.

*Garcinia, another herb with hunger-decreasing traits, may be useful in temporary weight management.

*Guarana, an amazon herb that contains high amounts of caffeine. I never use it.

*Gymnestra syl. Lowers sugar levels and may be useful in diabetes, not necessarily for weight loss. Increases insulin production. Repairs pancreatic beta cells.

*Bitter melon lowers blood sugar levels. It has side effects of abdominal pain and diarrhea such that I don't use it currently.

*Cinnamon. Improves diabetic control of sugar levels.

*Capsaicin. Thought to decrease appetite and increase metabolic rate.

*Fenugreek seeds have hypoglycemic effects.

*Banaba Leaf. Regulates blood sugar and insulin. Transports glucose into cells.

*Chicory decreases sugar levels.

*Licorice increases adrenal gland function and has been used for weight loss. Do not use if hypertensive.

*Caralluma Fimbriata, An herb that has been studied for weight loss with some success, origin in India.

*Pseudoephedrine is more a nutritional supplement that acts like a stimulant and can raise blood pressure. I never use it.

*Nicotine (tobacco) curbs appetite. Never recommended due to well-known health damage it causes.

*"Adaptogenic" herbs that may help ease stress levels are rhodiola rosea, eleutherococcus, schizandra, green tea extract, aloe, bladderwrack and kelp.

*Green tea. An herb I do not use because of the caffeine content, extractions are possible.

*Resveratrol at 200 mg a day may be useful for lowering sugar levels.

*Pokeweed and mistletoe may also be of value in weight loss.

*White kidney bean extract may reduce the digestion of starches. I don't use it.

Though herbs are generally considered safe for certain types of problems, they change our physiology and our thinking in subtle ways. Licorice, for example, is an herb commonly used as a sweetener and as an adrenal stimulant and thus it is associated with weight loss and added to diet bars. But licorice can also raise blood pressure. Ultimately, whatever an herb is compensating for is something

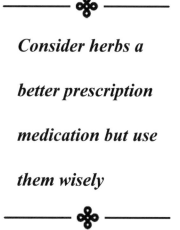

Consider herbs a better prescription medication but use them wisely

that we as individuals eventually must mentally and emotionally do by ourselves. Still, there are valid uses for many herbs in several health situations. Herbs are more natural than prescription medications but haven't got the studies behind them that modern science prefers to use to evaluate them. History of use and logic are ways to interpret appropriate herbal use.

Bariatric Surgery and Medications

I never recommend bariatric surgery, which involves "tier 5" procedures such as stomach stapling, roux-en-y, lapband or other surgical means to limit the amount of food your stomach can hold. One in 50 people die from gastric bypass surgery and its complications within one month using current surgical statistics. The benefits of stomach surgery come at a high risk, and you still need to deal with the inner reasons for being overweight. The only need for surgery I recommend is for those who are overweight and lose enough body mass requiring the removal of loose skin. Such plastic surgery is necessary to remove excess skin for both function and aesthetics.

Nor do I recommend any synthetic medication to deal with what are ultimately psychological causes for becoming overweight. Medications used in weight loss are phenteramine, phendimetrazine, diethylproprion, bontril and orlistat. At best, they should be considered temporary and I never prescribe them.

Human chorionic gonadotropin (Hcg) is an injectable drug that has been reported to be useful for weight loss. No studies have shown it beneficial over calorie reduction by itself however. Some reports indicate that hcg does reduce the sensation of hunger, making sticking to a low calorie diet easier. Fasting after 2 to 5 days also results in a loss of appetite or reduced hunger. The bottom line is that any drug cannot be continued indefinitely and thus everyone returns to their ultimate reasons for gaining weight unless they change their emotional and mental basis for overeating. I would not use hcg for weight loss.

Medications that *cause* weight gain are insulin, avandia, most diabetic medications except metformin and glucophage, steroids, benadryl, hytrin, cardura, minipress, inderal, topral, lopressor, tenormin, anti-depressants, antipsychotics, depakote, tegretol and neurontin. Find alternatives from your doctor when possible when you think you need these types of medications.

Laboratory Testing

What are your own bodily needs and how is your body functioning? I recommend getting blood tests for thyroid function, which are TSH, T-4 and free T3. I also recommend blood testing to check your metabolic panel, CBC, lipid panel, Hemoglobin A1C and urine analysis. Other blood tests you may need are C-reactive protein useful for inflammation, interleukin 6 and fibrinogen which may all be useful tests. Your doctor will know which specific tests to order.

Hemoglobin A1C is becoming the diabetes test best for monitoring health parameters. Many overweight people have diabetes or "pre-diabetic" metabolic syndrome that show increasing levels of Hgb A1C. A lowering of 1% of your Hgb A1C corresponds to a 21 percent decrease in diabetic complications. This should serve as motivation to many people to follow a vegetarian Paleolithic food regimen for their own health. In addition, if your initial laboratory tests are abnormal, your doctor may need special follow up tests like thyroid anti-bodies, cortisol levels, insulin levels and glucose challenge tests.

Detoxification and Health

While what we eat and supplement is important, so is what we "clean out."

Detoxifying is normal and a good thing. We produce substances that have to be detoxified or otherwise expelled from the body, even from normal eating and metabolism. On a cellular level, all cells of the body must detoxify constantly to maintain healthy functioning. Proper removal of wastes equals health and longevity for the cells, organs and body as a whole.

We have five main organ systems for detoxifying the body: bowel, skin, liver, kidneys and lungs. All these organs and systems do their part. Ideally, our bodies will purge the biggest portion of toxins through the colon. That is why having a freely flowing GI system is so important for moving waste out of your body.

Out with the old; in with the new. Since our intestines form the primary channel for most of our nutrition, it is always important to move the waste out of them. You normally should have a bowel movement within 10 to 30 minutes of eating a moderate sized meal and sometimes in the morning. That keeps your weight in balance. If you don't, you increase the exposure time of your body to colon wastes. This causes the other detoxification systems of your body, such as the liver, kidneys, skin and lungs to work harder than they should. This extra burden can manifest itself as altered energy levels, accelerated aging, and problems with the liver, gallbladder, lung and kidneys. If you chronically function at a dehydrated level and don't drink enough water, your colon motility can slow down to pull water back out of the stool contents. One of the physiologies that the colon provides is water re-absorption.

People usually think of bowel cleaning as meaning the colon alone, but the small bowel also can have flora changes and be in need of revitalization such as with probiotics. Good bacteria in your bowel actually produce essential nutrients for your body and are one reason that probiotics are sometimes given to re-colonize the bowel. The bowel does perform its functions in part because of its enormous surface area. The bowel has numerous "fingers" or projections called villi, which extend into the bowel lumen from the inside wall. These projections are like the fibers of a towel in that they increase the surface area of your bowel so that it is much more than a round muscular tube. In the same way that the surface area of a towel dries your body, the bowel's villi create a large surface area from which nutrient absorption takes place. Destroy this surface area with toxins, wrong bacteria, allergenic food reactions or debris and you greatly impede normal bowel nutrient interaction in your body.

Most people think the bowel is a one way tube of food to waste movement. However most of the peristaltic waves of the bowel originate from the hepatic flexure located in your upper right abdomen. Thus, your right side colon actually receives 90 percent of its peristaltic waves moving the opposite direction. The right side colon actually performs more mixing actions than simple propulsion of waste out of the body. Food wastes could theoretically stay trapped in this part of your colon for a lifetime.

There are many ways to return the colon to normal functioning, including using herbal teas, prunes, synthetic formulations, massage and stimulation of the abdomen and exercise. For most of us, hydration, exercise and dietary changes are usually enough to get things moving. However, people with long histories of constipation or consumption of unnatural foods may want to consider seeking out the help of someone who does colonic cleansing, ideally a very gentle and effective method of emptying the bowel. Herbal bowel cleaning uses a brush and sweep methodology using herbs that provide both functions. I recommend an herbal or hydrotherapy bowel cleanse if you have less than one bowel movement a day, a long history of constipation or are experiencing symptoms of toxicity.

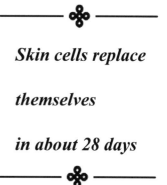

Skin cells replace

themselves

in about 28 days

The bentonite clay bowel cleanse has a long history of use and the ejuva cleanse is a newer popular form of herbal bowel cleansing. I have some concern about the aluminum content of bentonite clay and the sheer number of herbs used in the ejuva cleanse. At this point, both bowel cleanses seem to have more potential value than harm for some people who need to reset their bowel functioning. Everyone must keep in mind if you go back to old foods and habits then everything will return as before. So be sure you are manifesting new food choices and lifestyle to complement your physical therapies for better health.

Many toxins also leave your body through the skin. Your skin is an organ that produces metabolites. The skin enzymatically changes fatty acids and is responsible for vitamin D3 formation. The high number of skin allergic reactions shows just how active skin really is. Fortunately, many waste metabolites can exit through the skin by sweating which is one element of the traditional use of a sweat lodge for purification. Since you also lose salts or electrolytes through the skin, you may need to take extra replacement salts if you sweat heavily. After you have developed a good sweat in the steam room, take your hands and push down on your skin as you slide your hands over your body. This will increase the ordinary amount of extraction from your skin.

The lungs are also a major detoxifier of the body. The most common "waste" of the body would be acid from normal metabolism and this is released in the form of carbon dioxide you breathe out. The lungs however, also have anti-oxidant defenses and are important in glutathione homeostasis. Glutathione is naturally produced in the body to assist in the neutralization of harmful free radicals which can cause cancer. These enzymatic pathways in your body are important because they are active in cellular protection.

The liver is probably thought of as the most important detoxifier of the body, and metabolically, it probably is. The liver is responsible for phase one and phase two chemical detoxifications and is why liver detoxification and overall functioning is so important. It is also why taking pharmaceutical medications or excessive herbs can be strenuous or even dangerous to your liver. The statin drugs must be monitored for liver damage. The unnatural medications taken in by the body are primarily broken down and prepared for excretion by the liver. That is why you can have abnormally elevated liver enzymes in your blood tests when you are taking statin drugs to lower cholesterol.

The liver works much harder when the chemical input becomes less natural. It's also why alcohol consumption is so deadly for your body because in constant or large usage, alcohol excess overburdens the liver and destroys the liver cells, leading to cirrhosis. With liver dysfunction, you can have dark liver skin spots and excess metabolites backing up into your other cellular functions along with vascular abnormalities.

The kidneys are responsible for excretion of nitrogen waste products from protein metabolism and other water-soluble chemicals. Many synthetic drugs are excreted by the kidneys either wholly or after being restructured by the liver. It is the higher nitrogen excretion of high protein diets that can stress the kidneys and cause kidney dysfunction in people with borderline kidney problems.

Normally, all of our body systems have functional reserves. When we overburden our elimination and detoxification systems, dramatic and even fatal changes begin to happen to our bodies. Thus, taking any synthetic medication or consuming any stressful food in abnormally high quantities calls for careful consideration. Moderation is one of the keys to good health.

Nutrition is a tier one food therapy and is always the best place to start with an illness of body or mind, being sure that the body is getting the correct nutrients. First, this means food. Second, it means nutrient supplementation. Next we can consider the use of herbs. Pay particular attention to the original emotional and mental cause--an invisible emotional trauma in someone's life that finally manifested illness in their body.

Before significant problems occur in the body, people will almost always have subtle symptoms of pain or alteration. Western medicine laboratory testing and X-rays can give us physical information when things really get bad. But understanding and balancing a person before they get to the physical stage of illness manifestation can make life so much easier. You can read a lot of information about specific herbs on the internet, but you probably need to consult an herbalist and health practitioner for safety and appropriateness of herbal solutions.

When I do detox, I consider the main organs or group of organs involved. There are many potential detoxifying herbs and remedies as well as energetic/holistic approaches to detoxification. When I use herbs for cleansing with clients, I use them in a relatively safe but high dose and I pace through them by not giving them all at once. There are numerous purifiers such as garlic and the additional blood purifiers yucca, cinnamon, astralgus and burdock that we can use. These are just some of the useful herbs that Mother Earth has placed on all of the continents in amazing variety. Other herbal treatments require multiple herbs such as the ones used in Chinese and ayurvedic medicine. Consult an herbalist, a naturopath or a holistic doctor for their suggestions.

Fat cells are involved in more than storing fat. Fat cells are actually endocrine organs that relate to inflammation and various cancers. Fats are entwined with sugar metabolism and complex neurohormonal regulation. While sugars consumed can be converted to fat in fat cells, most sugar eaten (75 percent) is actually used in skeletal muscles. Insulin resistance increases with too much sugar use and, as a result, obesity partially increases. Cold increases the hormone adiponctin which increases insulin sensitivity and decreases obesity. Stress decreases adiponctin levels and increases obesity. Cold therapy in theory should improve metabolic rate and obesity parameters. Reducing core body temperatures may be an interesting potential therapy of the future to increase one's metabolic rate.

Stress increases cortisol which increases hunger and saves fat at the center of the abdomen. This abdominal fat is stored in the greater and lesser omentum. This type of weight gain is the usual type of stress-dependent weight gain you see in America.

Inflammation should be a target of treatment for overweight people and diabetics. This is why anti-inflammatory diets and hypoallergenic food choices are preferred for diabetics. Omega 9 essential fatty acid is anti-inflammatory and can be supplemented.

A modified vegetarian Paleolithic food plan, minus potential individual allergenic foods like the nightshade family, tends to be a very good anti-inflammatory hypoallergenic food regimen because it excludes the two most common food allergens that create inflammation: cow dairy and gluten.

I recommend nutrient-dense foods consisting of vegetables and fruit and occasional lean meat. I prefer raw food or use the cooked grains of quinoa and amaranth. I do not use dairy products from cows or wheat/gluten foods. If you can, find the best book on food preparation and cookbooks that show you how to get flavor and satisfaction from a low-carb and low-fat food plan. However, I would suggest that reasonable portions of pasta, potatoes and fattier meats can be eaten if you have a day that's been very active or involves greater exercise, if you desire. Not everyone can jump to a raw food diet, some people need cooked food, and individual variety will always be important for people.

Low-fat vegetarian diets such as this have been successful at reversing severe coronary artery disease mortality in people. Cholesterol, LDL, lung cancer and colon cancer are all decreased with these foods.

Chemically, foods range from acidic to alkaline. Better health results from emphasizing the foods on the alkaline side of the scale because they balance the metabolism of foods into acids. Normally the body can handle any natural combination. Remember: The mostly acid waste by-products of food metabolism are excreted by the various organs of our body. The lungs breathe out carbon dioxide. The kidneys release acidic to alkaline urine--whatever it takes to balance our internal chemistry. Too much acid, however, stresses the kidneys which have limits as to how much acid they can handle.

While glucose is usually thought to be the primary fuel of the body, you might be surprised to know that the preferred fuel for the heart muscles is medium-chained fatty acids. The heart can also use ketones and glucose.

Another special organ, the brain, prefers glucose. It too knows how to use ketones for energy and is also able to burn pyruvate and lactate. Fructose seems to be an old evolutionary sugar as the body possesses many biochemical ways of using fructose. Like our modern technological society, all the cells of the body have alternate fuel sources. High fructose corn syrup however, today has an added risk of the corn contaminants such as atrazine, a potent herbicide that some people believe is toxic--even as low as one part to a billion. Sugar in general should be avoided, but fructose derived from corn syrup has an added potential risk of contamination.

For the most part, drinks made with sugar and water (sodas, orange juice and almost all popular beverages) only go back about 40-50 years. Where in nature would you ever find anything like them? If you drink a liquid sugar drink, your body rapidly absorbs a huge amount of sugar, hitting your blood stream with sudden energy and a short term high. Unfortunately, your body responds by doing a couple of bad things. Since it recognizes the intake as excessive, it starts converting some of the sugar into fat. Also, the body shuts down its natural hormonal means of producing its own sugar, discouraging the insulin and glucagon hormonal systems from doing their work in the future. Recent scientific studies have shown that high sugar levels actually kill the insulin producing islet cells of the pancreas. When the intense effects of the sugar drop off, you feel a comparative lack of energy, and in varying degrees, your mind set becomes depressed.

Reacting to those feelings, many people simply drink another soda, further shocking the body into a false feeling of satisfaction until it wears off once again. Sometimes people repeat this cycle all day until they eat some solid food for balance or go to sleep, fatigued and exhausted. When people do this regularly for 20 years or more, they end up with diabetes, poor adrenal function, poor attention span, worse eating habits, drug and alcohol addictions, obesity or kidney failure.

Is there a viable sugar source? Use stevia sparingly for sweetening if you need to because unlike synthetic aspartame and saccharin, it is a natural sweetener and probably safer. You can also use non-corn derived fructose because it is sweeter than sucrose and you need less of it for taste. Agave is a source of fructose with a lower glycemic index than other sugars, but not a big help for weight loss. Overall though, you need to wean yourself away from any high sugar use to have ideal health and stable moods. This will start with taking a good look at why you feel the need to eat sugar. What energy or emotional problem are you compensating for by the heavily mood-affecting intake of sugar?

There are better options. Drink properly mineralized water, the most wonderful beverage of all, or substitute club soda or carbonated water for soda pop if you want a carbonated buzz. You can actually peel and eat that orange, instead of relying on some factory worker to squeeze 20 oranges into a cardboard carton for you. You can use almond milk instead of cow milk if you want any milk-like product at all and it tastes quite good. All in all, improving your eating means learning a few things. Learn to be more informed about what food labels tell you. Learn to prepare tasty foods without relying on sugar, salt and butter to make it happen. It will take time, but so would any other new lifestyle. Spices

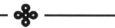

Sugar in liquid drinks, candy and desserts is the most deadly toxin in America for both kids and adults

can augment your food preparation and reduce the need for added salt. Spices such as curry, oregano, paprika, parsley, pepper, tarragon, basil, dill or basil can all improve the tastes of dishes so experiment. Your future health years are going to depend on your actions that you take now. These Outside-In changes are important for weight loss.

Elimination Diets and Toxic Food

You have a unique genetic body. Routine genetic blood tests will soon be standard medical testing. You may not be able to digest or assimilate certain foods, and don't know why. Food is more than food—there's a mental-emotional-physical connection and that mind-body link is a two-way street of communication. When you eat food that's not right for your body, you may experience a host of physical, emotional and mental symptoms that range from difficulty concentrating to body aches, to feeling drowsy, to becoming anxious, irritated or gassy. Yet, we're often driven to eat the very foods with which we have stimulating emotional associations (comfort foods, buttery cakes, pork rinds) even if the result of eating that food is damaging or harmful.

Eating mood altering comfort foods may initially feel good but later create bodily symptoms of feeling bloated, heavy, sleepy or anxious, thus adversely affecting your mind. Because of these physical distractions, it will be more difficult for you to concentrate on making innermost changes that can keep you on the road to losing weight. So if you have any of these symptoms, determine which food causes them. Remove these foods or additives from your house. You will have improved your health and ability to focus. To help you along, a hypoallergenic food regimen may help you initially when you are trying new food groups and losing weight. Eating only foods that maintain an even mood will benefit your weight loss discipline.

An entire area of holistic medicine concerns itself with what some people label "toxic food syndrome." It comes from eating foods that are not compatible with your individual body. Long ago, you would live on the same land that your forefathers lived on and eat the foods native to that area, just as your ancestors did before you were born. In conjoint evolution, your body and the locally inhabiting plants evolved together and this food that you ate would have been natural for you to digest.

In the modern world you probably don't live anywhere near where your distant relatives did. And you eat foods from all over the world without regard to season. Many of these foods are not compatible with your DNA, but unfortunately you don't know which ones they are. This incompatibility can lead to chronic internal food fighting, hyper immune responses that can eventually cause immune system compromise or complete environmental allergic over-activity.

In other words your body can spend a lot of its energy fighting internal abnormal food particles, and sometimes the body can turn on itself. The fix for this is to only eat foods compatible for your body or try a *hypoallergenic diet.* You can test for your individual incompatible foods by plain old trial and error. Compatible foods feel okay and cause no alteration to your mood or body function. Wrong foods will cause some kind of reaction, often a runny nose or noticeably faster heart beat after the first few bites. If you have eaten only one food and you get bloated, have gas, nausea, diarrhea, stomach cramps or excess mucous, it's likely that you and that food do not get along. Incompatible

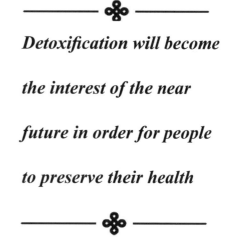

Detoxification will become the interest of the near future in order for people to preserve their health

foods can also make you feel weak or hyper and anxious. You might even get a rash or have irritable bowel syndrome or be diagnosed with gluten allergy in a traditional doctor's office. But to know for sure if a food is adversely affecting you, you can narrow the list of suspects by first using an elimination diet.

Elimination diets remove most products from your table. The end of a fast, for example, offers the ultimate opportunity for an elimination food regimen because you have excluded almost everything for an extended time while fasting anyway. Start with a few core foods you know you can eat without a problem. Commonly compatible or hypoallergenic foods include rice, banana, apple, potato, almond milk, chicken and non-citrus herbal teas. Then slowly expand the list of foods you eat adding one new food every two days to see if it causes any reactions. When you eliminate incompatible foods, you save a lot of energy and allow your immune system and digestive systems to heal and recuperate. You allow your body to function at its best state.

Foods that are commonly allergenic and should probably be avoided first by most people are wheat and other grains since most of them contain gluten. Peanuts, cow dairy products, strawberries and many other berries also tend to be problem foods. Citrus and exotic foods are also commonly allergenic. Test them on your body to determine if you can tolerate them or not. Nausea in the morning (reflux, GERD, ulcers) can mean wrong food consumed the night before, eating too late or more stressful emotions the day before.

Once you find what works for your body, eat those compatible foods and avoid those that are incompatible with your system. In your choices to eat, or after a fast, try eating foods native to the place of your ancestry. Makes sense! A reminder: Foods that I consider best for anyone with diabetes, metabolic syndrome or anyone experiencing inflammatory problems are basically a vegetarian, Paleolithic, no added sugar food regimen. Alkaline foods are preferable to highly acidic foods and tend to be more present in this food regimen. This means no cow dairy, gluten, alcohol, or any drinks except water and mild teas.

When you live in a state where your body is used to incompatible foods, you stay in physical turmoil over a lifetime and have a hard time telling your emotions apart from the effects of bad food. In the end, you can develop a food guide tailored to you that you can consider when you shop and when you eat out.

Yes, you can improve your moods and your willpower by eliminating sugar, caffeine and other stimulants and depressants. You can also improve your weight by supplying essential nutrients and using herbs conservatively and temporarily. A 5% loss of body weight improves glucose levels, insulin sensitivity and lipid profiles.

Cortisol is the recovery hormone your body makes after a life challenge, where it stacks and stores the energy of excitement. When you're conflicted or at war, through perceived mental challenges and emotional stress, initially you have constant high cortisol levels building up in your body. The problem is, it is out of balance with the reality - a sort of neuro-hormonal entanglement.

Once you get into that "Cushingnoid" big body, of course you're going to have physical, emotional-mental neuro-hormonal imbalance! What came first will be hard to define: overeating, cortisol or adrenal insufficiency. You're going to be mildly depressed, beginning insulin resistant --you're going to be hyper responsive to immune and inflammatory conditions. You're going to have the beginnings of sugar cravings or carbohydrate desires. You'll feel weaker.

Once stressed, it is harder to put on muscle mass. Thus it is very important to increase your pleasure and enthusiasm to improve your body. Making better food choices and converting fat to muscle, you'll resolve adverse symptoms and be in that lean body mass state of mind - a natural high that anorexics and exercise bulemics have in excess.

Like ayurvedic medicine and Chinese medicine have implied all along, all things and food have information encoded within them, their personality of sorts. It also says that how we feel, for example stressed or happy, can affect the response from the food after we eat it. Therefore, being happy, blissful or prayerful all affect food and how our bodies respond to that food that results in health or extra weight.

Welcome to a new life of enlightenment.

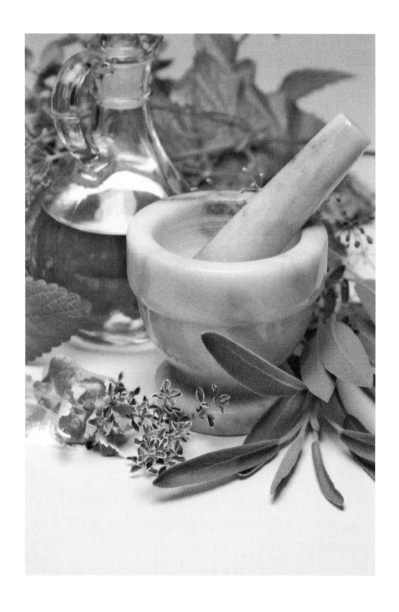

Chapter Eight

Ayurvedic Practices and the Benefits of Fasting

The food guide that I use the most is based on the principles of ayurvedic medicine. This 5000 year old medical and health system considers how all of life has characteristics of consciousness (~thought), energy and mass. You, the individual, will have unique tendencies toward thought, energy and mass. Foods have different characteristics of these same traits. If you are a high-thought person then you will have a "vata" disposition. If you have a fiery energetic personality then you will have a high "pitta" disposition. If you have a sedentary lifestyle and are overweight, then you have a high "kapha" disposition.

The key is to *balance* your personal constitution with the foods you consume or possibly the herbs you take. Each specific food and how it is prepared and eaten makes it increase or decrease these characteristics of vata, pitta and kapha in you. While this is a simplistic definition of ayurvedic foods, it may be something you would like to investigate as you develop your new personal food choices.

You can have mixtures of these three traits--vata, pitta and kapha--such that you might be just a vata personality or you might be a low vata, high pitta, high kapha person as it relates to your disposition, personality and body. If you are already a high vata person and you eat foods like dried fruits, cranberries, celery and peanuts (which are vata increasing foods), you will have even more racing thoughts and movement. Stress is a vata stimulating effect. Similarly if you are overweight and you eat foods like watermelon, coconut, potatoes, wheat, beef, salt and dairy you will increase your kapha even more and gain more mass as these foods make kapha higher or worse.

The key to ayurveda, as with everything in life, is balance, including your personal disposition. If you are a fiery person with a lot of anger or emotionality, then you are most likely a high pitta person and should eat foods that will tend to create balance. For you, eating foods like figs, grapes, sweet fruits, acorn squash, cabbage, cooked oats, turkey, lima beans and using wintergreen will help you.

Foods that balance or decrease kapha mass would be foods like apples, mangos, asparagus, peas, dry oats, rabbit, mustard and onions. Whereas foods that would increase mass ayurvedically speaking would be foods like oranges, sweet, juicy or heavy vegetables, wheat, beef, kidney beans and soy sauce. Along with this, overweight or high kapha disposition people should avoid eating between six and 10 p.m. The best times to eat are between 10 a.m. and 1 p.m, and again before 6 p.m.

When you are stressed, you're having vata increasing influences. To balance this, you can eat foods that tend to lower vata or use any of the herbals such as Perfect Peace tea. The same applies to kapha and weight issues. For example, experiencing higher stress vata situations tends to make you crave salt which is a grounding, kapha-increasing element. From an ayurvedic standpoint, the high stress (vata) nature of today's society has caused people to seek more grounding. Most foods that tend to lower or balance vata also increase body mass (kapha). This might explain in part how our high stress world has led to a need to increase grounding which a larger body mass tends to do.

With ayurvedic principles, you can use food to give yourself the most balance and, therefore, control to your body, thoughts and emotion. The classifying of food lists is ancient. While I recommend ayurvedic food lists, once again, your unique food compatibilities matter the most. You need to combine all this information with your personal choices such as eating vegetarian or preferring to eat some meat. Make the modern day choice to avoid unnatural foods and excess sugars.

While all pitta foods and spices may tend to increase metabolic rate, I do not include pitta foods in the "golden food" list for a specific reason. The number of people with GERD symptoms would all be made potentially worse if everyone turned to eating high pitta spicy foods. For that reason they are left off the golden food list.

Foods Beneficial for Reducing Weight and Stress

There are very few phytonutrient foods that both decrease kapha (weight) and decrease stress (vata). These are the few "golden foods" that can help you with weight loss and stress:

*Fruits: apricots, all berries, cherries, peaches, ripe mangoes, soaked raisins, strawberries, kiwi, lemons, limes and some grapes.

*Vegetables: artichoke, asparagus, bean sprouts, red beets, sweet carrots, daikon radish, fenugreek greens, cooked garlic, well-cooked green beans, horseradish, cooked leeks, mache, cooked okra, cooked onions, radish, cooked shallots, crook-neck yellow squash, scallopini squash, summer squash, watercress and zucchini.

*Grains: amaranth, some cooked oats, basmati rice and wheat bran, if you have no gluten allergy.

*Legumes and nuts: soaked and well-cooked legumes, aduki beans, red lentils, tepary beans, hot tofu and tur dal. Nuts that are beneficial are well-soaked almonds.

*Seeds: chia, flax, sunflower and pumpkin seeds.

*If you use sweeteners, then apple and pear fruit juice concentrates would be best.

*Condiments that are beneficial are black pepper, coriander leaves, daikon radish and all radishes, lettuce, mint leaves, mustard and cooked onions.

*Spices are generally very useful and include ajwan, allspice, anise, asafetida, basil, bay leaf, black pepper, caraway, cardamon, cayenne, celery seed, cinnamon, cloves, coriander, cumin, dill, fennel, fenugreek, garlic, ginger, horseradish, mace, marjoram, mint, mustard seeds, orange peel, oregano, paprika, parsley, peppermint, pippali, poppy seeds, rosemary, rose water, saffron, sage, savory, spearmint, star anise, tarragon, thyme, turmeric, vanilla and wintergreen.

*Animal foods that would be better for you are poached eggs, some turkey and some chicken.

*Beneficial dairy include fresh goat's milk, fresh yogurt and ghee, which is clarified butter.

*The beneficial oils are cold-pressed safflower oil and white mustard oil.

*Teas: ajwan, basil, catnip, chamomile, cinnamon, cloves, ginseng, hawthorn, juniper berries, lavender, lemon balm, lemon grass, orange peel, osha, pennyroyal, peppermint, raspberry, rose flowers, saffron, sage, sasparilla, sassafras and wild ginger.

*Greens: Spirulina and blue-green algae would be beneficial.

I believe in eliminating virtually all sugar-containing beverages for optimum health. If you do occasionally have beverages, those that would be better are aloe vera juice, apricot juice, berry juice, carrot juice, carrot-ginger juice, cherry juice, hot-spiced goat milk, grape juice, mango juice, peach nectar and low-salt vegetable bouillon.

Conversely, there are foods that should be avoided because they are particularly aggravating to kapha (weight) and vata (often stress). They are watermelon, dried fruit, frozen fruit and any fruit with sugar. Pickled vegetables are bad as are spaghetti squash and tomatoes. Don't eat cold cereal. Aggravating meats are beef, lamb, pork and venison. Legumes to avoid are kidney beans, common lentils, soy beans, soy flour, soy powder, soy margarine and tempeh. Nuts to avoid are peanuts. Seeds to avoid are psyllium. Don't use white sugar. Don't use ketchup. Don't use almond extract, tamarind, amchoor and neem leaves. Avoid all dairy, hard cheese, cow's milk, ice cream and sour cream. Avoid all deep-fried oils, rancid oils and breaded products. Do not have carbonated drinks, cold dairy products, icy cold drinks, alcohol and tomato juice. Also, avoid chlorella.

Even your own mental state when you are preparing food will impact the quality of your food, and so will your state of mind as you eat it. The ancient caution to eat good food and "not from an enemy" still holds true today. That biblical writer was not referring to poison or he would have pointedly used that word. It meant that the intent of the person preparing food has a real effect on the consumer's health. Thus, there might be some very real reason why mom's chicken soup really did taste best and got us healthy! The life and energy put into foods exists on other wavelengths that can affect your health. This same principle even applies to the water that we drink and the quality of life given to the animals that we raise.

If you accept that your thoughts affect the quality of your food, you might try giving a blessing over the food. Stopping to give thanks helps slow down overeating and balances eating for immediate pleasure. As you experiment with holistic nutrition and occasional fasting you will begin to notice the evenness of your moods. That comes from removing the harmful foods from your food regimen. You will notice an improvement in your health from giving your body the essential vitamins, trace minerals and essential fatty acids it has been needing. You will notice the joy of having even moods by avoiding the disturbing foods.

As you start to shift the direction of your health for the better, emotional prosperity can come along as the next car on your train to good balance. When you search for and drive out the food demons and defects of your own ill health, you make room for the blessings and grace of your own unique divine nature which will come forward and fill your presence with its beauty. These things will never come from a fast-food chain, an alcoholic drink, a chocolate bar or any sugar-filled beverage bottle, despite what the commercials tell you. In fact, they've been blocking too many of us for years. All you have to do is take the first steps that lead to true freedom-- freedom from want, freedom from ill health, freedom to eat what you want in moderation and real freedom to be happy.

Dieting vs. Fasting

Fasting can be a mysterious event to some people since it involves, basically, stopping the routine eating of meals for a set time. Fasting can provide a means to cure a host of ills. But who fasts and why?

In proper fasting, you put your mind to work contemplating your thoughts and emotional drives. You take in no substantial food and I suggest you mildly supplement with essential nutrients and some amino acids. Dieting is body focused and food focused. Fasting is more mental, emotional, and spiritually focused with an eye to causation of how you live. So concentrating on a diet actually magnifies food drives because you're adding to your mental food lists of things to do and eat. It's why proper fasting works--there are no food thoughts or menus to prepare, so you eliminate the build up of mental lists of what to eat next. Fasting is better for working on the mind.

A fast is not necessary for everyone. When you establish your correct foods and lifestyle, you can lose weight without going on a fast. Prolonged fasting will tend to lower your metabolic rate and it will not add muscle. However, fasting can augment your changing as it detoxes your mind as well as your emotions and your body. Fasting gives your GI system a rest and eliminates food allergy problems for the length of the fast. What improvements you make by not eating harmful foods increases your willpower and clarity. You can tackle bigger issues which are going to be about your emotional drives, thoughts and beliefs. After a successful fast you can rev and tone your body with the trio of healthy uncontaminated food, exercise and a clear mind.

Medical science considers fasting a natural phenomenon and bodily function. The body has been metabolically equipped by nature to go long times without food. All animals will fast to heal. Look to nature, because it is showing you what works best. Great informed people of history have used fasting for physical, mental and emotional well-being.

What I have added to fasting is a modern day capability to monitor your fast more safely than previously possible. You can lose one to two pounds per day by fasting and supplementing with a low-calorie nutrient mix augmented with amino acids. To keep your metabolic rate from going lower

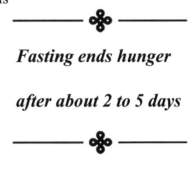

Fasting ends hunger

after about 2 to 5 days

you must stay physically active during this time and reinvigorate with exercise afterwards.

Fasting with Intention

Remember that what your body takes in during a fast will be more highly absorbed. For example, trace minerals will be highly absorbed during a fast. Conversely, watch out that you don't put inferior products into your body during your fast that would be nutritionally harmful.

Fasting is the most natural way to lose weight. The body has numerous physiological responses to fasting that will make you lose excess weight. Always fast with water, electrolytes, some nutrient and amino acid supplementation and always fast with intention to discover yourself and change.

Fasting creates the ketone process of fat removal with greater intensity than any diet. Since fasting is inherently short term and done without high protein or fat consumption, it doesn't overload your kidneys or other organs. In fact, fasting gives your digestive organs a rest. Most of the body switches over to reserve methods of energy consumption and production. Fasting allows you the time and intensified focus to experience how you really function, often uncovering hidden or deeper drives within you. Fasting breaks the routine lifestyle of living and allows you to bare your mind's beliefs and drives for examination.

Prior to a fast, it might be good to have a colonic cleansing and empty out the old waste products that may have been in your bowel for years. I recommend this if you have had a history of constipation or toxicity.

Specific organ detoxifications may prove useful after the initial cleansing work of some fasts. I have had patients with long term chronic elevated liver function tests return to normal after using nutritional and herbal liver supplements that detoxify and heal the liver. I have had patients with gray hair grow back their original color after using nutritional and detoxifying treatment methods to their health.

During a fast, I nourish myself with a small amount of blended natural food. Mostly I use re-hydrated prunes, apricots and figs. You could probably choose many natural low calorie amino acid foods if they are bland, natural and compatible for your body. But I also blend a raw apple and a banana. The banana is probably the most foreign food that I use, but it adds a good tasting creamy texture to the drink. To this I add spirulina, a nutritious life force sea algae powder, also thought to be a stem cell enhancer. Once blended, I keep this liquid in the refrigerator and use only a few teaspoons at a time during a 24 hour period. You can blend in whatever foods you like as long as they do not upset your stomach. I like the prunes because they tend to make the bowels work--a plus for most people.

Prebiotics, which are basically fiber or fructooligosaccharides act as substrate in the bowel to promote the growth of friendly bacteria.

You always have bacteria in your bowel. You have more friendly bacteria than friends. But you can also have unfriendly bacteria, particularly when you are sick. Prebiotics help the friendlies by making the colon chemically a better environment for them. Natural fruit and vegetables also provide fiber for your bowel and friendly bacteria.

You can use probiotic bacteria to re-colonize your bowel with more friendly bacteria. We have identified many species of these friendly bacteria. The following are "good" bacteria: Lactobacillus rhamnosus, L. acidophilus, L. plantarum, L. salivarius, L. reuteri, L. casei, L. bulgaricus, acidophilus DDS-1, L. sporogenes, Bifidobacterium bifidum, B. infantis, B. longum, Streptococcus thermnophilus and Bacillus laterosporus. I also use Saccharomyces boulardii. Friendly bacteria help break down your food and make nutritional cofactors that your body then absorbs. They do not produce toxins like harmful bacteria.

Bio-chemically, your body switches to producing and using ketones during a fast. Ketones come from breaking down fat, and you can easily test for ketones in your urine with testing strips called "chemstrips." Testing your urine is easy and will tell you just how much you are in the fat breakdown mode.

Your body's stamina and your monitoring abilities improve with each fast. I fasted intermittently over six months before ever doing a fast over one week in length. During this time of intermittent fasting, I cleaned up my body, improved my eating and working lifestyle and started to become more aware of my emotions and thought processes. I gained experience with how my body fasted and became confident in my monitoring techniques for hydration.

I developed the nutrient supplement that worked best for me to provide some amino acids to my body every day along with vitamins and essential co-factors. I also pre-fasted by supplementing my body with all the essential nutrients, natural vitamin E and the essential fatty acids before doing any fasting. *You don't want to fast with a depleted nutrient state or depleted anti-oxidant state in your body.* Loading up with essential nutrients before fasting allows your body to detoxify safely.

During a fast you will burn up your fat reserves. In these toxic times, this becomes complicated by fat-soluble neurotoxins. Because neurotoxins such as pesticides, insecticides and herbicides that may have gotten into your body are stored in fat, they will be unlocked, released and re-circulated when you break down fat. The detoxifying organs of your body will then attempt to metabolize them and excrete them. Because fasting accelerates detoxification of unhealthy parts of your body, you will want to be well-loaded with the anti-oxidants such as natural vitamin E and its co-contributors vitamin C, selenium and zinc. There are other herbs that help purify and detoxify the body, but I prefer to use them away from a fast in separate treatments.

Some doctors would associate ketones with ketoacidosis. Ketoacidosis can be a problem for diabetics when they produce ketones and have impaired insulin functioning. During fasting however, ketosis formation is a safe and natural physiological adaptation. After 24 hours of fasting, your liver runs out of glycogen and begins to break down fat, producing ketones and acetyl coenzyme A which are used by most of your cells for energy. Some glucose is formed by breaking down protein in the liver for red blood cells and the brain, so it is wise to have some amino acid intake during fasting. The liver makes more ketones which can substitute for some of the amino acids needed by the body so that after seven to ten days of fasting, the body requires fewer amino acids. Ketones are thus very healthy and helpful, especially when you know they are being taken from your fat stores.

Your body protects against muscle loss by using more fats and ketones. In addition, your kidneys excrete more ammonia as compared to urea, creating a more balanced adjustment to the fasting state. The ammonia excretion balances the acid/base concern for fasting. *It's good to transition in and out of the fasting state slowly.* Your body can safely adjust to a fast, as long as you take adequate amounts of vitamins, minerals, water and some amino acids. After a fast, you will be able to build up your muscles in a better health and state of internal body purity.

You may even discover your original fasting with intention becomes much more than the reasons for which you started. It is at the core of fasting that you occupy yourself with matters of the heart and mind. So when you fast, pay attention to your being and focus in with one single goal of understanding yourself, one drive at a time.

Fasting vividly brings to your consciousness the means and reasons for your drives, feelings and thoughts. As these invisible mechanisms relate to your weight or overeating or under exercising, examining them will be key to losing and then maintaining weight.

Fasting can lead to euphoria that strengthens the body and mind

During a fast, as in normal living, the body has a constant need for amino acids. If you don't eat them the body will break down some of its own muscle to get them. When fasting, the liquid supplement I prepare contains amino acids for the body during a fast. If you want to avoid or slow down potential muscle loss during a fast, I suggest light exercise and being sure to have some amino acids throughout the day.

You can project a goal, question or state of being during a fast. You can increase your understanding and awareness of others and the outside world. You can intensify your understanding and communication with your inner self during a fast. You can use the fast to monitor, change and manipulate your dreams, goals and real life. Fasting automatically provides detoxification of your body but it also allows detoxification of our mind and emotions if you want to direct it there.

Whenever you stop the basic routine day to day functioning from fasting, you allow an opportunity for hidden realities to come forth. Those hidden realities may be how you waste your time in life, what distractions you have been allowing yourself or what "problems" you have been experiencing.

If you lack understanding, fast for it and seek clarification and options. Your mind is quite powerful. You can develop greater comprehension. A fast should always be done with a positive mental attitude. Allow yourself what naturally may come up and ponder it, process it but you should always come out of it with an enthusiastic and positive state of being. Keep that in mind. You should resurrect good self feelings and resolve issues for the better future. You can change from pessimism to optimism during a fast and understand depression and anger that may reside within you.

Fasting naturally increases growth hormone during a fast. A certain euphoria can come from fasting. Internal energy actually goes up during a fast.

I use fasting as a combined psychological and physical means to identify mental and emotional defeating patterns while losing physical weight. Ketosis improves hypertension, cholesterol, diabetes, and suppresses hunger. Besides the amino acids, you also need 30-70 gm carbohydrate a day and 64 ounces of water a day. You also need 1 gram of salt a day which you can get from mineral supplements, vegetable juice or two bouillon cubes.

Each person has his or her own set of ideas, issues, emotional and mental states that could be improved upon. You can intensify prayer during a fast and dedicate that time along with the food that would have been consumed to the nourishment of others. *So if you have a problem, fast on it.*

No fasting should be done if you suffer from cardiac disease, catabolic health states, e.g. infection, are post surgical, have cancer, syncope or dehydration issues. Fasting is not for growing adults or children. If you ever become negative during a fast or unable to stop thinking about food, then you need to come out of the fast. Fasting must always be done in a positive state of mind.

There are many types of fasts: no water, drinking water but no food, juice fasting, and specific food type fasting. I don't recommend any of these for various health and nutrient reasons, particularly juice fasting due to the high liquid sugar concentration of these fluids.

Preparing For Fasting

By now you should have used the nutritional information in this book to shift your eating pattern toward natural, sugar-free, caffeine-free foods. You don't want to have to deal with the effects of coffee, sugar, or caffeine addictions or other types of imbalances during your fast. These types of problems should be addressed before considering a fast.

Before you begin, there are a few items you'll need to purchase or make sure you have on hand.

*The urine Chemstrips "SG" to test the specific gravity of your urine as well as to determine when the glycogen stores in your liver have been used up. These are sold at pharmacies and will allow you to check the concentration of your urine to determine whether or not you are properly hydrated. If your urine is too concentrated (the instructions will tell you how to determine this) you need to drink more fluids.

*A journal in which to record your thoughts and your dreams during your fast. Your dreams at this time can be very revealing if you know how to interpret them. Mary Summer Rain's book *20,000 Dreams* can help you to figure this out, or else you can simply record your thoughts, emotions and experiences. Looking at them later can reveal a lot about what your subconscious is telling you or experiencing.

*Supplements including high-quality basic nutrients, minerals, trace minerals, certain detox formulas can work and a high quality amino acid supplement.

*I prefer to use club soda instead of vegetable juice because of the bicarbonate, but I add potassium, magnesium and zinc to the bicarbonate which is in club soda. Six-ounce cans of vegetable juice to be used sparingly for electrolyte replacement may also be used.

*High quality pure water with minerals.

Beginning Your Fast

Although you may be dealing with negative issues for a reason, the overall philosophy of your fast and your mood must be positive. You are trying to investigate and change yourself. The fast will give you greater clarity to do that.

Start by doing one-day fasts.

One-day fasts will introduce you to both the monitoring and the initial effects of a fast. Keep yourself well hydrated and take a high-quality vitamin but no other supplements. Keep your mind on positive things and try not to think about food or your mind will rebound after the fast. If you catch yourself thinking about food, take control of your mind and do any of the contemplative exercises or emotional energy exercises previously listed.

Contemplation is the mental technique most useful when beginning fasts. Give yourself one issue to contemplate for the day. After completing three-to-five one-day fasts, you can go on to do three-day fasts.

Three-day Fasts

The best time to do a three-day fast is on a long weekend when you can start on a Friday and devote time to yourself. Make sure you have no other obligations during this time and that you can be primarily alone. To do this, you may have to plan your fast well in advance.

Fasting is primarily a solitary journey of self-discovery. A friend who is a good sounding board may be helpful during this time of contemplation and evaluation of your beliefs and emotional habits.

Fasting puts your pancreas and insulin systems to rest. Diabetics can fast but they must monitor their sugar levels very closely. The need for insulin will be markedly decreased if not unnecessary when fasting.

While You Are Fasting:

*Each time you urinate, check your urine for specific gravity. Drink six-to-eight 12-ounce glasses of water each day.

*Urine Chemstrips will show that you are ketoning, an indication that your body is burning fat for energy.

*Take the vitamin and mineral supplements mentioned before.

Using Protein Supplement Mixtures

You can use this option to help supply essential vitamins and amino acids during your fast:

Place about eight pitted prunes, dried apricots, and dried figs in an eight-ounce glass (enough to fill the glass to the top).

Fill the glass with water and allow the fruit to soak in the refrigerator for 12-to-24 hours. Transfer the re-hydrated fruit and it's liquid to a blender and add a half teaspoon of Spirulina and six tablespoons of a high-quality non-dairy, non-gluten protein supplement, one cut up banana and one cut up apple. Blend until smooth.

Keep the mixture in the refrigerator and sip it intermittently throughout your fast. Fasting for three days gives you the time to deeply contemplate specific issues you want to become more aware of in your life. You can use any of the contemplative suggestions and emotional exercises to help you do this. Your greater mind will answer your specific questions when you contemplate thoroughly.

Longer Fasts

After you've completed three-to-six three-day fasts you can begin to fast for one week and then eventually two weeks. I do not advise fasting for longer than two weeks, but fasting is such a personal experience you will have to judge for yourself. Never fast longer than what makes you feel comfortable and safe.

As in all things, you can overdo it. Be sure to give yourself healthy food breaks between fasting episodes to fortify your body with the essential fatty acids and nutrients it requires for health. I recommend you take at least as much time off between fasts as the number of days you are fasting.

The more you fast, the better your body becomes at it. That's why you repeat many shorter fasts before going on to longer ones. Your ability to monitor your fast for dehydration will improve as you become more familiar with your body's functioning.

People commonly hit a three-day emotional wall that makes day three of a fast feel challenging. It can bring up all sorts of feelings, but if you work with them, ultimately, you'll gain greater clarity about some of your issues. Maintain your positive consciousness and press forward with your mental contemplations and emotional exercises. You may be experiencing your thought processes and emotional tendencies full-on and objectively for the first time.

If you are fasting to lose weight, it is essential that you contemplate the thoughts, emotions, and lifestyle choices that have led you to overeat, not exercise, and so on. You need to determine how you handle stress and pleasure and discover the origins of your lifestyle choices. This is the true purpose of fasting: to find, alter, and balance your deepest beliefs, thought processes, and emotional responses. By doing this, you will purify and bolster your will, faith, conviction, and consciousness. It is an ultimate *Inside* technique to help you along.

What to Do to Enhance Your Fast

Keep your body in some sort of motion, as it's meant to be, by using a few of these techniques.

Full-body massage can do wonders to help you release the tension from your body. During a fast in particular, you may experience great emotional release just from having your body massaged. This is because your elevated consciousness causes a heightened tendency toward energy-release.

Stretching keeps the circulation going, aids in flexibility and feels good. This exercise takes 15-to-30 minutes and is particularly good to do in the morning. Be patient to not stretch to the point of pain. If you do feel a painful spot during a stretch, breathe deeply into the area and relax as you exhale. Think about what you need to release from that particular area of your body. You may be surprised what specific thoughts come to you. As you exhale, affirm that you are thankful for any experiences in your past that have

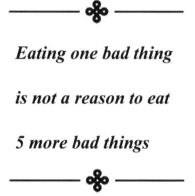

Eating one bad thing

is not a reason to eat

5 more bad things

allowed you to be more loving, more sensitive, and more open. Then visualize the pain leaving your body along with the experience.

Ending Your Fast

It is important to come out of a fast as if you had not been doing anything special at all. Your way of being should continue from fasting time to normal living time. Continue to be aware of your thoughts, and do not allow your mind to focus on food. You can control your thoughts by creating another subject for your mind to consider or by involving yourself in an activity or awareness that is not food-related. Increase the physical activity exercises and toning of your body to return to an improved natural state.

The day after your fast you should consume mainly liquids and soft foods. When you begin to add other foods back into your diet, they should be light and preferably vegetarian. If you are ready to dive into a steak, you've probably got a lot more to contemplate.

When you reenter everyday life you will probably notice, where you didn't before, challenges to the discoveries you made during the fast. Almost everyone around you will have a tendency to want to keep you the way you were before in terms of your eating, lifestyle, and personality. Don't give in to others when they want less for you. This can be more or less of a challenge, depending upon your home and work relationships. You should be happy that you're making strides toward managing your weight and your life. Self-talk and affirmations will help you to continue on your forward journey.

Consider that it has taken a lifetime for you to get this way. You should be patient in realizing that a few months is nothing in terms of reversing old patterns when you give it your attention.

Right Thoughts,

Right Food,

Right Exercise

Right Lifestyle

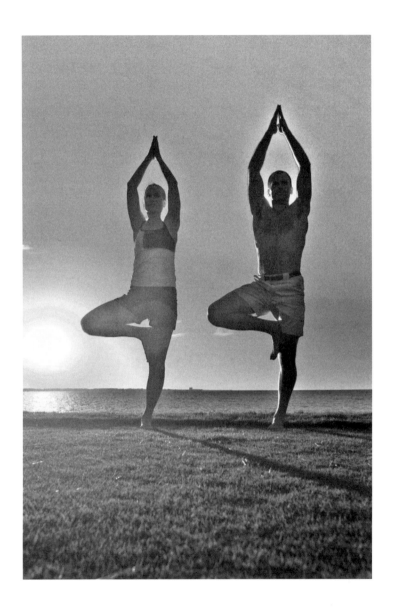

Chapter Nine

Exercise - Getting Fit and Motivated

Compared to the essential nature of food, exercise is probably more important in maintaining a proper weight than is the food you eat, though both are necessary. Physical activity or the lack thereof, is the most linked lifestyle leading to being overweight, illness and death. No matter what you do, some exercise or physical activity is going to be necessary to lose weight and keep it off. When you stop using your body, biochemical changes occur that work against your health.

Breaking Through Negative Attitudes About Exercise

The reasons people don't exercise relate primarily to these two emotional and mental perspectives:

•People view exercise as work and as something negative and therefore don't do it.

•People don't exercise because they believe they don't have *time,* cannot find the time or they do not *make* the time.

When you don't have time in your life to do the necessary and fun things to stay healthy, you are out of balance in your mental and emotional realities.

Most people's early experience with exercise goes back to their elementary or high school days of physical education (PE) and their participation in sports. Sports were often seen as something requiring very hard labor and a competitive mindset which many people identify as either too much work, or "not who they are." Since participation in many of these sports programs was challenging, many people view exercise as a conflict where they judge themselves. Also, many people's early experience with exercise was competitive and threatening, where there were more "losers" than winner's rewards. These inner beliefs are still active for many people and they discourage themselves from exercise without even knowing why.

Exercise has many benefits: The only way to burn more calories during a day is to be more active, which for today's culture means setting up a regular daily and weekly schedule of physical activity. The best way to increase your calorie expenditure via your individual metabolic rate is to put on muscle mass. Muscles burn more calories than other tissues even when you're doing "nothing." The more calories you burn, the more food you can eat without worry of gaining weight. If you enjoy eating, which you should, then you need to put on the muscle.

There's another aspect to why people are exercise-averse. They often identify the panting and straining of physical exercises as tiring, draining and negative. And there are the typical "side effects" of exercising--the perspiring and the sensation of tighter, pumped muscles. Afterwards, people smell bad and have to take time to shower and clean up, which they also think of as another time-consuming irritation. My experience is that most overweight people hold these counter-productive if not self-destructive beliefs about exercise. Shopping—in supermarkets or malls, though, is often the only way people who need to exercise will get out and move!

Breaking the negative "Inside" attitudes you have toward exercise is crucial to maintaining what needs to be a lifelong habit of pleasurable physical activity.

For exercise setbacks, motivate yourself! On a piece of paper, list the benefits of exercise, strength training and walking versus continuing as you are. For example, you gain energy and strength rather than continuing on feeling sluggish and out of shape. Reviewing this comparison list will inspire you to rethink what you want out of life. The simple truth is that you need to retrain your mind to alter self-sabotaging habits and increase the awareness of your body by enjoying its sensations.

As an example, let me tell you about a patient of mine, a woman I'll call Laura, and examine her experience with exercise:

Laura accomplished great success with healthy food choices and a balanced general lifestyle. She looked normal but her percent body fat was over 30 percent. She was also very intelligent. Her last internal challenge was to deal with her negative attitudes about exercise which she did not know she had. Laura always believed herself to be "not an exercise person," and "uninterested" in physical activities. Like so many people, her reasons to back away from exercise were more meaningful.

Growing up, she had early imprints of exercise as something negative that were originated during her peer-pressured school years. Laura had to change this deeply-held view of exercise being distasteful to finally master her body. She needed to enjoy her body during and after exercise, the sensations it brought and to develop the mental view of exercise as freeing and fun. Important too, was for her to re-calibrate her sense of having time to exercise. It took a few months, but she triumphed over old and useless beliefs and took up a sensible exercise routine.

As with Laura, the concept of "no time for exercise," are words you often hear from people who sincerely believe it. Even if you run or walk from your home, it requires at least 30 minutes of your time to get dressed, exercise, and maybe shower afterwards. However, the *concept* of having no time goes even deeper and usually comes on after your mid-20s. People have often been instilled with a "get ahead" psychological work drive, sure that they've "got to sacrifice to succeed and make money" which would then put everything else in perspective. They believe money will make them feel better. They believe that success is the priority.

Having "no time" goes hand-in-hand with perceiving life from the vantage point of being about degrees of stress. If you don't really have time, then you are overworked and/or channel all your energy into making money. This doesn't leave you enough time to participate in physical activities that are healthy. "Having no time" is another form of self-imposed stress.

Any possibility of finding a true balance between allowing your life to unfold peacefully and having to maintain your body with physical activity gets buried. If this sounds like you, "having no time" needs to be traced back to when you first became so busy and pressured in life. These reasons will be specific to you. Correcting these self concepts in your own mind is essential for health and maintenance of proper weight through physical exercise.

If this is you, at some point in time (in your history) you made a decision that led to living stressfully. Identifying this in your memory can help release it. If you don't release your underlying wrong beliefs, they will keep driving you in the direction you've been going.

Another reason people don't exercise is that they blame the gym or workout location for not having what they want. One seriously overweight client told me that her favorite cross-training machine, located in the basement gym of her apartment building, was broken. Therefore, she could not exercise. That there are probably a dozen other locations near her house for her to find such a machine will not enter her consciousness. Her belief is that for her to exercise, it must be convenient and provide the one piece of equipment she likes, or else, she's back eating chocolate instead. She was looking for reasons not to exercise. Flexibility, as an inner trait, would help this person.

It is very useful to have like-minded friends to assist you especially in exercise, since everyone has moments when a friend's enthusiasm will ignite your own and carry you forward on days where you just give up. Social exercise can be more enjoyable for some people.

There is another mixed reason for some people not exercising and that's because:

•**Some people, after physical activity and/or exertion, complain about being "sore."** When you are highly stressed, increasing the body sensations becomes too much for some people, and they feel more aware of negative stress than the benefits of movement. Not only does exercise help you maintain weight, but exercise heightens body awareness. Body awareness is a good thing, but for people who are already too stressed and agitated, "feeling sore" becomes "feeling pain" and a very negative association for them.

Muscles have memories too, and you need to build up flexibility and strength. You need to expect some degree of body soreness or increased body sensation when you are exercising. In fact, that feeling of soreness is usually natural muscle growth. If you find yourself thinking that you'd rather opt out of exercising rather than deal with natural body changes, you need to examine what doing nothing does for you! If you have a negative attitude about exercise, soreness will become pain. If you have a positive body concept, soreness will more likely become fulfilling as you exercise because you know you are improving and your body is more capable. Attitude!

Be smart about your routines. Pushing yourself to do more at the gym, or jogging another few miles, for example, or rushing to get into shape *can* lead to outright pain. You must start small and go slowly as you increase the limits of your physical exercise routine. You must have patience to go for the long term health benefits and not hurt yourself by taking on too much physical activity or muscle growth too soon. Exercise should never become something you do "to just get over it."

You have to make exercise a game and enjoyable activity.

The addition of these emotional and psychological insights about not exercising is directly correlated to why you gain weight and remain overweight. Understanding and curing these psychological blocks and how to accomplish this, is at the heart of *The Inside-Outside Diet.*

Examine these elements to get you going:

*Look at the exercise routine that you may be avoiding, or not doing your best to incorporate into your schedule. What is stopping you?

*Be clear about whether you've neglected exercising out of old negative ideas that its work and that you'll never like it, no matter how good it is for you.

*Ask yourself if you have given up exercise with the excuse that you have no time--if it is a self-imposed shortage of time, real or otherwise.

By identifying these *Inside* elements of emotional distress as it relates to exercise, you will know where to refine your search for what is happening in your emotional life and how to fix it.

Understanding What Exercise Does For You

The equation for energy expended while walking or running goes like this: (calories burned) exercise work = force X distance. What this means is that you spend roughly the same calories walking two miles in one hour as someone who runs two miles in 10 minutes. So take your time and start walking. It is better just to finish the distance as far as exercise calories goes. 3500 calories = 1 pound of body mass. You spend about 100 calories for each mile you walk.

Physical activity necessary for survival in older civilizations is still necessary today in the form of elective exercise. It's an evolutionary requirement for having a body that functions optimally and in good health. No one exercise is complete by itself unless it offers muscle resistance, enhanced heart-lung breathing, blood circulation and strengthens the finer balance, spatial relationship and eye-hand coordination. Necessary work that often satisfied much of these in the past has to be made up with intentional exercise of today. I envision community work efforts in the future being done in part for physical health.

In the area of exercise, you need to be engaged in cardio-pulmonary activity such as running, treadmill, bicycling, swimming or anything that gets your heart and lungs moving blood at an accelerated rate. This cardio-pulmonary activity is also called aerobic conditioning and triggers blood flow through all parts of your body activating metabolic pathways to burn calories. It increases metabolic rate and stimulates growth hormone which will increase your lean body mass (muscle) to fat ratio. Some studies indicate running long distance or greater than 30 minutes causes people to lose muscle mass. This is why distance runners need to interval train or cross train with strength exercises to stimulate lean muscle mass formation.

You need to apply muscle conditioning in the form of resistance training to be in best shape. This puts an increased load upon your muscles stimulating them to increase in size while also stimulating your bones to remain strong (countering osteoporosis).

There are so many studies coming out that modify the recommendations for how to exercise that I leave the subject at this time open to later interpretation. Still, there are some basic recommendations that you can use. Always warm up with gentle walking or movement before starting a more vigorous portion of your exercise. This can include a gentle stretch and a cardio type of movement. After the main part of your physical routine, do some stretching again as your muscles are warmed and more capable of gentle stretching. After exercise, this kind of gentle touching stretch can also discharge any static energy tightness that may have come on from the exercise itself.

In strength training, to gain muscle mass you need to do repetitions at the weight and number that end in muscle fatigue, where you can't do any more. This signals the body to make more of those muscles and builds them up bigger and stronger. Consuming healthy nutrients immediately after your workout may be more beneficial for building up the strength of your body than delaying eating. Essential amino acids stimulate muscle growth more than non-essential amino acids.

The easiest thing for most people to do is to start walking. If you're very overweight or out of shape, have a doctor check your health first. If you or your family have a history of cardiac disease, then you also need to be medically approved for any exercise program. Even simple walking should be done with a gradual increase of duration. Other robust exercise is desirable but be sure of your cardiac health prior to starting any exercise program. Becoming short of breath, having chest pain or feeling faint are sure signs to see a doctor. Other symptoms are excessive sweating, nausea or pain in your arms, neck or jaw. Still, most people can start walking for exercise. Make it enjoyable so that you look forward to it.

The most important thing to say about exercising is to make it positive and rewarding for yourself so that you continue to do it. First, think that you can exercise wherever you live, walking down the road or street. You can do push-ups and sit-ups or jumping jacks in your own home. You have to make it enjoyable which for some, will require re-setting your mind about how you think of exercise or how you think of your body. Setting goals for how far and how much exercise you do will give your mind focus and drive to attain it.

To be motivated to exercise and keep fit, you have to enjoy your body, what you can do with it and the sensations it can bring. In the morning, don't think you have to be locked into the idea of only working out at the health club or that you need special equipment. After your morning drink of water and your mild activity, you can do sit-ups, leg raises, push-ups, jumping jacks--old style calisthenics basically. I still jump rope as an aerobic exercise. You need to get your body toned and moving. This will get your lymphatics moving after a night of sedentary activity. Keep exercise new, refreshing and exciting. Variety will help, so change your exercise every month to keep it stimulating.

Getting Rid of that Belly

There is some indication that consuming the types of fat called monosaturated fats that are found in nuts may be healthier in terms of not putting on the omentum type of body fat. That means internal belly fat. These would be the main fats you would get in a vegetarian Paleolithic diet where there is no cow dairy or animal meat. Avocados and seeds also have healthier fats.

Getting rid of that belly is often the hardest and the last thing that you will have to accomplish. To have a flat abdomen without fat requires a few things. First, know that sit-ups alone will not do it. Sit-ups strengthen the abdominal muscles which is good but has very little to do with inner omentum abdominal fat. Losing that fat will require total body energy expenditures through exercise with reduced calories over a long period of time. Toning your abdomen will then create that final look. Fasting is one of the few ways to accelerate fat loss enough to drop a percentage of the body fat to lose that belly. And then afterwards, an aggressive exercise program with healthy vegetarian raw food would be the best way to create that trim abdominal core. Aggressive exercise without fasting will accomplish a lean abdominal core but it will require more time spent in exercise than most people are willing to allocate.

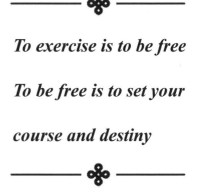

To exercise is to be free

To be free is to set your

course and destiny

Exercise that creates a toned abdomen is particularly useful for getting rid of that belly fat. Belly fat is of two kinds: subcutaneous fat outside the abdominal wall and fat within the abdominal wall stored in your greater and lesser omentum. Removing this latter kind of fat is the most difficult. I've found the exercises that create tone in your abdomen, such as running, jump-rope or trampoline exercises develop abdominal wall tone which seems to improve the removal of that abdominal fat.

Morning really is the best time to exercise. There are less distractions or interruptions. Exercising in the morning allows you to get energized before losing the desire in your day from other obligations. You have the clearest mind in the morning and therefore the best effort. The body's abilities come from the mind being the clearest to exert willpower and to exude emotions that are purest.

The next best time to exercise is in the early evening after work where you can rid yourself of any excess tension energy created throughout the day. You can run it out of your body and get your body moving the same time. Discharging evening energy will give you the best sleep too as a side benefit. Running, like many exercises, can be a meditation in itself. For your own self-discipline, keep in mind that discontinuing exercise is the first health habit to fail when you're faced with stress or extreme boredom. **Stopping exercise is the first sign of someone beginning to fall off a weight loss program.** Don't start skipping exercise you have set up unless you have a replacement physical activity.

The Daily Plan to Stay Fit

Incorporate this plan as a way to keep on a schedule that you both honor and enjoy! Start to notice your body more when you exercise. Your increased awareness of your body sensations can bring you more enjoyment during and after your exercise and bring you into more conscious awareness.

*To kick off your Exercise Plan, take walks or exercise in the morning or early evening, or both. On a weekly basis, take longer walks, run, swim, train with weights, nature walk or play tennis. Weight lifting types of work-outs can be done two times a week for maintenance and running or jogging could be done once or twice a week. Whatever you enjoy should be the most important guide. Plan to exercise on the same day of each week as structure may support you.

*If you're traveling, there's no excuse to not exercise. Try these on the road tricks: pack your running shoes and GPS running device. Don't travel to excess so you have no time to exercise or eat healthily. Plan your work schedule with *living* in mind. Plan ahead where you stay. Use a cooler in the car to pack healthy foods such as apples, bananas and healthy water. Do not patronize any fast-food establishments. While they have gotten better with their food choices, they still cater to that "lack of time" mentality which is still a fat/sodium/sugar trap. Don't drive until exhaustion hits you.

*Holding your day together will hold your life together. Conversely, letting things go one day may let your get-healthy plan slide into chaos and stop your life-saving changes. People often blame work as the reason they have to drop their exercise. Your healthy life is more important than your work. Be tenacious and firm with yourself and honor your commitment to your body.

You should do 5 to 10 minutes of light stretching or light exercise when you first get up and after you drink some water. Hold your stretches for 30 seconds to 2 minutes so they are relaxing. A short outdoor, fresh air walk would be ideal. Starting out peacefully in the morning should be a priority habit.

Daily activity should be done in a non-stressful environment. Curtail your work situation for a focused, non-distracted amount of time. Take breaks from your work to refresh your mind. A mid day walk trumps a mid day coffee, donut, or margarita. Having too much to do can lower the capability for any meaningful work to be done. Dumping stress with exercise or with mental clearing exercises will prevent you from dumping stress through excess harmful eating.

Wait to eat in the morning until you first feel a little hunger. It's not as important that you have breakfast as it is crucial that you not wait until you're famished or you will overeat and eat without control of food choices. Eat light and vegetarian the first part of the day. Committing to this will allow your meals to be more planned and be of a higher quality.

If you have high glycemic foods (sugary foods) they should not be eaten in large quantities first in a meal. Most vegetarian foods will be high fiber, which are good for your bowel's motility. Low calorie, raw, nutrient-dense foods are better than empty high starch or high fat foods. Drink fresh mineralized water throughout the day. If you snack, alternate natural fruit or vegetables--no liquid drinks of any type except water. Look to the "golden food group" I listed earlier for better food choices to lose and maintain your weight. Your afternoon meal should be the largest meal in terms of calories and fat/protein.

Remember that on days when you exercise, you could eat more. The game of healthy body weight versus being overweight is derived simply as a ratio of how much you work out divided by how much you eat in calories. So on days you exercise, you allow yourself to eat more if you want. On days that you aren't active, stay light and vegetarian with your meals. This gives you a balancing plan for weight versus activity to keep your body weight in check. On days that you are very physically active you may eat higher glycemic-load foods like pasta, rice and potatoes.

If you are prone to hypoglycemia or mood swings, then you need to avoid sugary foods altogether, or high-glycemic index foods, except for at the end of meals. Having no caffeine, MSG or any herbal stimulants will be particularly important for you.

Whenever you shower, end the shower by turning the water temperature to a cooler setting. Cooler temperatures reset your internal thermometer for higher basal metabolic rate functioning. Also never use a steam room or sauna more than once a week unless you are doing a specific detoxification plan that emphasizes this treatment for a while. Keeping a cooler feeling around your body may generate a higher metabolic rate.

<u>Your Personal Trainer</u>

If I could assign a personal trainer to everyone who wanted to lose weight, you would lose weight. The personal trainer would remind you of your goals daily. A good personal trainer would smile at you, say nice things to you and encourage you. They would be a presence in your life and a scheduler of your time.

Because of this presence you would make it a priority. You wouldn't ignore someone standing there beside you trying to help.

You are - can be your own personal trainer. You should be saying nice things about yourself, giving time and presence to your goal. You would be there to say how meaningless food indulgences are. You would tell yourself when you're ready to binge that you really are just not happy and motivate yourself to change. Be there to give you a massage and take stress away. Say nurturing things to yourself. **This personal trainer is you!** You should be reminding, encouraging and prioritizing; staying on course. Can you be this way to yourself?

Hire a personal trainer if you can afford one, hire yourself and perform for yourself. Think of that 2 hour time block between 5 and 7 pm, your trainer, your work-out, your dedication, your commitment, your success. Eventually you'll have the joy, drives and euphoria of any exercise and body enthusiast.

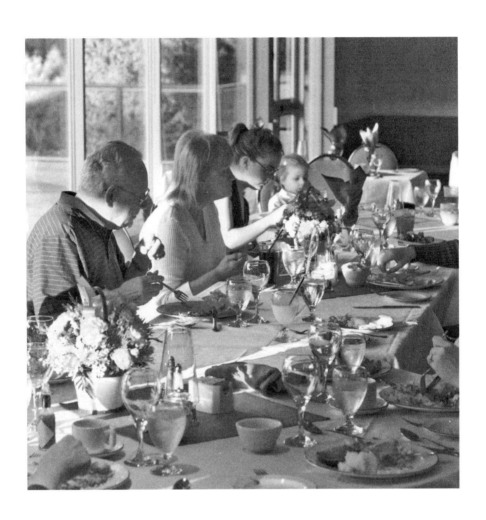

Part Four:

Culture, Hormones, Depression & More

Chapter Ten

Individual Insights to Health

Culture and Overeating

Modern culture makes it easy to get simple requirements like food and clothing, but our culture makes it harder to conquer emotional stress for ego development. People's thoughts are conflicted, emotions discombobulated and psychic energy strained. Many choices and more gadgets exist to speed everyone on. Self-management and self discipline are not taught. But, there are simple offerings of food readily available everywhere to lessen our wills, conviction, clarity, attention span and willpower. People seek a quick fix, quick tasty food and try not to deal with the stress of the complex arrangements of lifestyle. These are cultural problems.

Cultural mores are lifestyle elements that are different in various cultures, even within the United States. One's personal ethnic or local culture is an emotional issue that can be at the heart of becoming overweight. Cultural habits for some people exert great influences on how much you eat.

Maybe eating is the focus of social events, family events or even sporting events. Then, there are the marketers. Advertisers not only want you to be hungry, but they want to associate their food product with emotional relief, happiness and satisfaction. If you buy into their pitch, the result is excess calorie intake and excess weight. Be aware what your culture is promoting and you'll be more aware and empowered to know when you are being manipulated into overeating. Resist the subliminal overeating messages when you catch yourself being manipulated. Do you really need to have crispier chips to make your day?

This is classic cultural manipulation about food, "all you can eat buffets." They are not really healthy, and don't be drawn into them. "Free refills" of anything are not healthy. You have to remind yourself

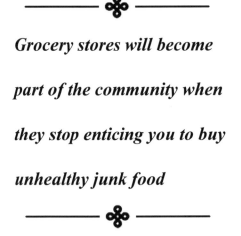

Grocery stores will become part of the community when they stop enticing you to buy unhealthy junk food

that these things play on your sense of a good deal. The cultural sense of "more is better" is a falsehood in terms of food, where <u>less</u> is better for you. In fact, studies of cultures where people live longer consistently show that these people eat less calories than other unhealthier people. You have to be more correct and smarter about your health than the culture you live in. The bottom line is that you just have to say NO to the advertising!

You need to be particularly aware of the candy, chips and soda pop impulse sale products almost always set up in check-out lines or next to the cash register, from gasoline stations to almost every type of business, especially grocery stores. These displays are done for one purpose only: to make money off your impulse buying. Don't let yourself be the victim of others' business manipulations. Keep in mind that any store that locates these products at their check-out stands is not looking to do you or your children any health favors, but are only reaching into your pocket for their personal gain. Any business owner that truly cared about you or your children would not place these items in these locations or perhaps, even sell them at all.

At home, it's up to you! Say no to dessert, second helpings, rituals of coffee and donuts and being served the wrong kinds of food. Say no to meats if you are trying to be more vegetarian, no to cow dairy and gluten if you're trying to avoid these common allergens, no to heavily-fatty foods, too many sweets, ice cream and the like. You have to risk people being unhappy with you for awhile when you start to say no to what they want to serve you.

You need to change your perception of "sweet" from something rewarding to something that is harmful in the quantities that most people consume. No matter how much sugar you cut out of your food regimen, you will still be getting plenty from other sources. Think of your health and the example you set when you say no to harmful food choices and change your eating habits. Other people and your children will see what it's doing for you, and they will be influenced to do the same.

Peer pressure can help you or hurt you, but eventually, you need to do everything on your own. When you first encounter peer pressure that is harmful, you either say no to peer advice or no to the peers themselves. Find new friends who have your same goals and standards in mind. When you walk into a restaurant and wonder what the food is like, look at all the people eating there. If they don't look healthy, consider that the menu is based on foods that are wrong for you, and don't eat there. Ask your questions about the food and how it's prepared before ordering. I would like all restaurants to list the sources of their food and water on the back of their menus. To be healthy today, you need to know.

We often think of pleasure from food as a reward. This is confirmed by both our culture and families which have established a history of food rewards built into the thinking. We have the idea implanted within us from our early upbringing that cookies, candy, soda pop, desserts and sweets are "good" rewards. They are not "goodies," but "baddies," since sweets are not so sweet for our health. We need to change how we think about them in terms of what they really bring on--excess weight, diabetes, heart disease and other health problems. **Thinking correctly, leads to doing correctly.**

Dealing With Friends and Family

Friends and family may help or hinder you in your desire to lose weight. You need to say yes to what helps and no to what works against you. Speak up for your desires and let anyone around you who is trying to counter you know that you are improving your health. If friends and family try to undermine you despite telling them you want to lose weight and be healthier, then you will have major decisions in your life about the nature of the relationships and what they really mean to you.

Having a good friend who will remind you of your course for health and why you are losing weight and exercising can be very helpful, but you must eventually do it on your own. Groups can be helpful in maintaining weight in the beginning. You don't want to make a cult of weight loss that is always reminding you of food, however. You have to be able to hold your positivism and self-discipline when you are most stressed, most challenged and conflicted in life.

Because we are social creatures and have needs for companionship and pleasure, we tend to want to be around people. When those people have poor food choices like any other habit, we will tend to do what they do, giving yourself reasons to do the harmful things in your life just to be with them. So while you are in transition to a better structure of your mind and daily lifestyle, you may need to re-structure your friends as well. Don't let your need for companionship become an excuse to eat poorly.

Decrease conflict with other people as it increases stress. This change in how you interact with others will help you immensely. Give everyone a place to exist and believe they will not hurt you. Feel secure in yourself and that you deserve to be happy. Be appreciative of good relationships and what people give you and what you give in return. This minimizes stress.

Use emotion-stabilizing exercises to re-group. Relax, let yourself be sensually more alive, and most of all, consciously allow yourself to change.

Modern society presents us with so many difficult choices to make and obligations to keep, that sometimes our minds feel literally overloaded. *Mental overload* may, in fact, be one of the primary reasons we become overweight and out of shape. Interestingly enough, most of what's going on inside that causes us stress is self-generated. While you may think that your mind is working overtime because of issues in the outside world, the majority of those non-stop thoughts come from your ongoing effort to protect yourself from something that *might* happen. Worry is a problem you can't actually see or touch, but it is one of the most health-damaging aspects of modern society. **Worry counters willpower so stop doing harm to yourself.**

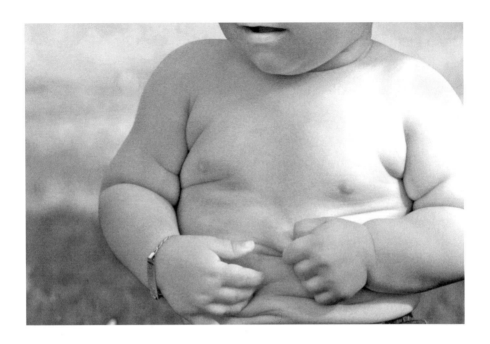

<u>Overweight Children</u>

Kids don't eat naturally on a three meal a day schedule. Children will easily skip a meal or snack, depending upon how they are raised. For children and growing adults, a small breakfast can be beneficial for development but it shouldn't be heavy in calories. Eating is a learned activity and in many cases, so is exercising—even for children. Some kids have to be coaxed into moving or participating in the simplest physical activity.

Happy, socialized, children at play often do not want to eat at all. Don't make eating the source of all joy, comfort and social interaction for your children. These essential emotional needs must be supplied apart from the influence of food. Otherwise, food can become identified with your children's emotional life which can manifest as overeating and weight problems later.

Overweight children have many of the same issues as adults except children are much more able to easily change concepts and activities.

Most children can change the influences that affect them more easily than do adults—but it will matter in what kind of environment they're being raised. Overweight parents more typically raise overweight children. But, being able to talk logically with children about their bodies, what happens to them if they overeat and why it's important to exercise and eat the right foods will make them more open to make changes.

By and large, children will do structured exercise and alter their food habits with greater ease than adults. Children's parents have the major influence on them when they're young. Home habits of eating, food kept in the kitchen, refrigerator and pantry are very important. The ability to keep children socially and physically active is often up to the motivation of their own parents. **Overweight children can be allowed to grow into their developing bodies without the need for dieting per se.** Children need to form their daily habits when they are younger. They will be influenced more by their peers than adults as they get older.

Fourteen percent of kids and teenagers are overweight. You can treat them with less restaurant eating, better home food and education when they are old enough. You need to treat the parents when treating kids for excessive weight. Decrease TV and video games and encourage outdoor activities. Remove all sugary drinks from the refrigerator. Say no to candy. Structure improves the minds of both children and adults to maintain good habits.

Overweight children get too many calories relative to the calories they expend in physical movement. Physical education was considered less important than regular classes in school and therefore reduced in participation, now it has come back to show its importance for health as more children are overweight than ever before.

I have a great concern for what the generation of "pacifier babies" will be carrying into adulthood. The constant satisfaction of our feelings by putting something in our mouths may be very damaging when as adults, stress is encountered. It seems almost all children today are controlled with food rewards. At some point we need to stop the early life mental and emotional implanting of this oral reflex to stress relief.

Women, Weight and Hormone Replacement

Many women struggle with excess weight at the menopause or perimenopause years. At this time of fluctuating hormone levels, maintaining peace and avoiding stress can be particularly challenging. Overeating is a common mechanism of emotional and mental distraction during this time.

Synthetic female hormone replacement of estrogen has been found to be unequivocally risky for women because studies have shown an increased risk of stroke, clots, heart attack, dementia and Alzheimer's. However, natural hormone replacement has not been fully tested for the same risks. Natural hormones are being used at this time for women who want relief of symptoms of menopause and are willing to accept a potential risk of their use.

The estrogen that declines with menopause actually has three types: estrone, estradiol and estriol. Estrogen decline is responsible for the hot flashes and mood swings. The progesterone that also declines seems to balance the estrogen and is also responsible for balancing mood swings. Balancing the moods with added progesterone may protect you from overeating episodes.

Other hormones such as testosterone, DHEA and cortisol all are involved in the menopause years as they interact with the other hormonal systems including your thyroid. Hormone testing is available from certain labs or your doctor if you want to check where your hormone levels are functioning. Besides the standard cortisol level urine test, another way of testing cortisol is the 4 times a day salivary method. Some people have ultra low cortisol in the evening with adrenal exhaustion.

Natural relief for perimenopausal symptoms is obtained from

exercise. A diet high in vegetables and fruits is also preferred. Broccoli, chick peas, cauliflower and cabbage all contain phytoestrogens which may be particularly helpful for menopausal women. Fermented soy may also be useful for menopausal women as a source of phytoestrogens. A balance of omega 3 and omega 6 essential fats may also improve your health and mood.

Other nutritional supplements, and in some cases, herbs may be able to give you some relief. For some women, gaining stability over their hormonal status improves their ability to avoid the urges to overeat. There are some herbs that may be used in lieu of prescription medication that will help your perimenopausal moods.

Black cohosh is an herb primarily used to stabilize hot flashes but also helps with mood swings. Chasteberry or vitex helps mood swings and hot flashes. Dong quai also helps. Evening primrose oil may also help with hot flashes. Red clover contains isoflavones like soy, and helps with hot flashes. Mood and energy stability is the goal to keep from overeating.

Depression and Weight

Many people who put on weight deal with depression. Every physical and mental step you make towards improving yourself will be a step towards getting over depression. People who are depressed about their weight were afflicted with other emotional management problems for some time before they became overweight. While depression due to health or being overweight is a current issue, it is also important to address your mental and emotional situation when originally you put on the weight. Something was operating at that time in your life that caused an eating for pleasure or eating for tension release lifestyle to ensue. Something stopped your joy pursuit in life.

Every person with depression will have an original cause, a thought or belief they have embedded within themselves sometime in their past. All people with depression will have one or more emotional reaction patterns they have imprinted in their psyche that makes them drive energy downward. All persons with depression are served some way by their depression, i.e. they are getting something out of it. This can be a control of energy levels, an opening or closing of vulnerability, or re-directing of emotional input from others.

No person has gotten out of depression by something or someone outside of themselves, unless the event was extreme. You have to look within yourself, self-talk and live within awareness to get out of depression. While simply trying to be positive may be helpful 90 percent of the time, at some point you have to search out negative circumstances and beliefs to find and reverse a depressive origin to your emotional state. The original cause of depression must be found for permanence of health. The *understanding* of your depression will free you to cognitively change yourself to living in the present.

There are consciousness techniques you can use to find and release depressive self beliefs associated with any event in life. There are also some food and nutritional therapies you can use to assist you in this correction and stabilization of mood. Prescription medications and herbal products such as sam-e and St. John's wort may be helpful to relieve depression but usually block the person from seeking the source of the underlying problem.

All depressed people have a reduced energy and censured vulnerability that is falsely protecting them somehow. What is unique today is that so many people can survive living at home without working, and by receiving medical disability, they can stay in protected depression for a lifetime. They are simply cheating themselves out of a good life!

The Real Cookie Jar

What was really in that Cookie Jar? We did not suddenly become overweight. Overeating is a learned trait. As enthusiastic and happy children, we'd usually not think about food. Also, we wouldn't usually stress for very long before it was released. We'd sleep fine and we did as our parents told - for good or for bad!

Somewhere along our lifespan, we became controlled – became controlling by food. Parents started it oftentimes. Cookies were good rewards, extra dessert and pacifiers of our emotions. As adults we began to self control and self medicate with food - all unconsciously. We did it from our memory, without thinking about what we were doing or the consequences. So now in this culture, where we've never been taught about ourselves or healthy food, and we tend to look outside of ourselves for the cause of our problems and our solutions, we're massively ill.

Now you can substitute anything you eat for "cookies" that is a fat gaining, energy disrupting, unhealthy food. You know cookies have nothing in them that are nutritionally helpful. You know they make you sick. Gas, stomach aches, bloated abdomen, heaviness, diabetes, cardiovascular problems, mood problems and weight gain all result. Yet we will knowingly eat what is bad for our health, mood and life longevity. Such is the power of beliefs and emotions.

What was really in those cookie jars? The answers: We need the love. We need the security. We need the pleasure. We need the stimulation. Emotionally and subconsciously, we need the "okay" feeling we get from eating them. Now you could add gasoline to that cookie and most people would still eat it. Why? Think about it! Can you get the emotional balance you need without eating it – yes you can!

Mental thoughts alone have little power. But couple a mental thought with an emotional feeling and tell yourself it is "good" and you ingrain a powerful reaction that drives you to repeat that activity over and over. For most people, their wrong cookie drives were implanted within them when they were a child. We were "told" the cookies were good. We were told they were a reward, were told they were something we couldn't have all the time, only on special good occasions so we wanted them even more. We were reinforced through a lifetime of repeated causes, stresses and rewards till we come to the age we are today, still eating cookies.

All of your cookie habits are just like that. Strong mislabeling of emotional rewards as solutions to problems, "owies," sadness, hurt, pain, boredom and whatever is ailing us. But the truth is all our emotional cookies are ailing us. They are perpetuating a culture and lifestyle of sickness. Our parents may have started the habits. We continue it. That's because we all want rewards and pleasures to distract us from our negative experiences to more positive ones.

When we're acutely in this disturbing eating state, all we know is it feels better than dealing with our problems, even if the problem exists within our mind. We can satisfy and generate secure, happy, emotional and mental states directly without reinforcing ourselves with foods that are temporary and really bad for us.

New thoughts by themselves are not as strong as old beliefs that are repeated with emotional significance. It doesn't even matter if the old beliefs were true, they often were not. We continue them. We remember vague feelings of "feeling better" after eating our cookies. Our simple mind holds imprints of solutions to all our negative emotions and all our missing positive emotions. Whatever behavior pattern was instilled in your first 20 years of life from childhood experience to your adult drug, food or addictive life experience, we continue as our cookies of today.

We have to start individually to fix this. We have to start with telling our self the truth which is: WE were WRONG! Some of the "good" things in our past were really not good at all. They were bad, harmful, physically sickening and emotionally misleading. They were not helpful. They numbed and made dumb our inherent intelligence. Like the apple in Eden, they led us astray into poorer decisions and worse health. So now that you are 35 % body fat or higher, at least 20 pounds overweight, walking around the house as your maximum nature experience, unhealthy, and *dying*, what are you going to do about your body and emotional health, your lost Eden, your lost healthy life?

Well, you've already started if you are motivated to become healthier. You realize something is wrong. *Why* you feel bad, tired and depressed you've been reading. Start to tell yourself the mature, adult, responsible truth.

Next, you start to take action on your adult knowledge. That knowledge has been poor, incomplete and misguided in the past in the form of diets and drugs previously used to mislead you from the truthful original cause of what happened in your life. You decide that you will be responsible and take over from where you are today.

First, add some peace and contentment to your life by taking the nutrients you may be lacking and start doing the emotional balancing exercises designed to get you immediately feeling better. You start to add walking for exercise and enjoyable relief.

Second, you start to drop all negative emotions you feel residing in you today using awareness and the emotional healing techniques described in *Start Living Stop Dying - 10 Steps to Natural Health*. That can take awhile. Third, you decide to put in some work and effort for your own survival. Fourth, you stay alert to your personal revealed causes and lifestyle mechanisms of why you are overweight that spill out of your beliefs and emotional patterns.

Furthermore, educate yourself about good foods. You start correctly eliminating food that is hurting you. Unplug yourself from that television that has been acting like an iron-lung machine artificially giving you life. The three hours of TV watching and snacking is no longer helping you but harming you. You pray or meditate mindfully for help and you do what is helpful. Eating naturally, healthier food is a start but it has no immediate strength of repetition with emotional reward, so plan on repeating good habits for one year for them to become a foundation and for you to become emotionally balanced.

When you are caught off guard and your personal demon cookies try to step in at moments you are feeling stressed or under satisfied, you confront the truth and self-talk yourself through the reality of health. **Use substitute and delay tactics to improve your food choices for health.**

Tricks and Small Things That Help

These are some small things and "tricks" you can do to promote a lifestyle of health, nutritious eating and a better weight. These can be very effective for change since we are often broadsided by unexpected encounters in life that tend to re-create old lifestyle habits.

*In car trips with people, talk, don't eat. Don't order supersized portions at roadside diners. Supersize is super bad. Downsizing is good! Change the concept.

*In general, drinking water before a meal will tend to make you more satisfied. Taking supplements when you feel hungry, with a large glass of water, can make you feel satisfied. Keep low calorie raw vegetables like celery or fruits in the refrigerator for when you want to have a snack. Alternating low calorie radishes, celery, kiwi or other vegetables and fruit can get you through weeks of snacks.

*A little protein and fat may help end snacking binges so keep almonds or Brazil nuts in your kitchen. For some people, this kind of snack curbs their appetite better than other foods.

*Slow down when eating meals and consciously chew and savor them more. This will give you better digestion and overall satisfaction. When you gobble down meals in a short time you never get the level of enjoyment you should have. Your brain will have time to hear your stomach.

*Meditate when you feel an abnormal drive to eat. Finding a peaceful life or creating a good feng shui environment in your home and work will contribute to your sense of peace and tend to counter negative stress energy in your life.

*Take a short nap in the mid-afternoon for 10-15 minutes. Whenever you sleep, you knock out the accumulated thoughts and emotional energies and thus balance your drives again. This may prevent the build up of emotional drives at the end of the day.

*Quit looking at the refrigerator as the answer to life's needs or for joy.

*Emptying the refrigerator and pantry of every bad ingredient and liquid drink except water is a must. Only shop at grocery stores using a list, and after eating dinner. Never buy food when you are hungry.

*Shut off your TV and invent a life. If you watch television where there are constant food commercials planting food thoughts into your consciousness, you'll be further stimulated to overeat. Constant barrage of food commercials and shock television can waylay your consciousness and willpower for accomplishing what you want to do in life. You can waste away all your free time in life by watching two hours of TV every night and your true pleasure will be under satisfied. Intentionally get out of the sedentary evening lifestyle where you go home, watch TV and usually eat while you are doing it.

*Always eat in the dining room. Do not eat in the bedroom or living room. Never eat after 7 p.m. and don't drink after 8 p.m. Make a plan and force your self to go out and do more social activities.

*Never eat the last of anything and instead, leave the last bite on the plate. You tell yourself you do not need anymore. "I am satisfied." This subconsciously affects your mental beliefs and programming that you are full, otherwise you get an unsatisfied alert that subconsciously gets stored in your mind.

*You need to have goals to assist you. You can make a physical goal, an emotional goal, a mental goal and a food goal. For exercise it may be to walk one mile, or it could be to swim 10 laps of a pool without stopping. Goals will tend to keep you on track and motivated.

*You need to make a clear mental and lifestyle demarcation between your previous life and your new life of health. In some cultures, you might be given a new name to signify a new you. You need to think of the old ways as the old days. **When deciding what to do, think of what the old you would do and then think of what the new you would do.**

*To set a change in your life, you can make some physical reminders. Change your clothes or the way your house looks. Place a photo that means something to you on your refrigerator or on your car steering wheel. Place every physical, mental, emotional and lifestyle goal somewhere visible. Something that positively reminds you of progressive goals that occupy space where you spend your time. Your home, your bed, your car and your work are the main locations. Placing reminders of your new goals will help you transition between the old and new you. Not that old feelings and temptations won't come up, but you'll be empowered from within and reminded from without.

*Other tricks can be commitments to no dessert or not eating out. For one, you'll have better, known food ingredients when you prepare at home.

*Make the decision not to eat cow dairy and remove ice cream from your refrigerator. **One at a time, find substitutes for every harmful food you eat.** For cow milk, substitute almond milk. Instead of margarine use whipped butter or ghee. Don't buy canola oil; use olive oil, sesame oil or sunflower oil (not for cooking). Forget forever about pop up toaster pastries and buy apples and bananas instead. Display them in a bowl on the table. Pasta, potatoes, rice, bread, breakfast grains (all can be used sometimes) can be replaced with leafy or green vegetables that can be cooked or eaten raw. Chocolate and candy snacks can be replaced by mangoes, blueberries, cherries or any natural fruit. Your water can be filtered.

*Meditate for 10 minutes to raise energy and develop peace.

Eating tension can be stabilized with daily meditation and a weekly de-tensing massage.

*Plan a job change if that's what matters to you and until you get out of that job, *change your perception of your job.*

*If you feel like eating out of boredom, do 40 sit-ups, 10 push-ups and 5 minutes of stretching followed by a walk. You can go inward or outward when you need to reset your affirmations to counter any negative food.

*People who bother or stress you out can be put in perspective immediately or over the long term, depending on your choices. Politely leave for a walk with deep breathing when stressed by someone. Remind yourself to maintain who you are and forgive others for their opinions or immaturity. Perhaps a sincere talk with them could be a solution. These types of personal issues will always need your personal decisions for the best resolution. **Disconnect the food-emotional issue connection.**

*Decide to master or educate yourself one healthy step at a time. You may want to read about Chi Gong and then take your first class. You may want to read and educate yourself about some form of physical activity and then go try it. Keeping reading material fresh in your mind about progressive healthy matters will keep you positive. For worry, you can use prayer or mediation. Major issues arising in your life can be handled by deep contemplation and time set aside for yourself to discover the origins and then solutions to the problem.

*Use club soda instead of soda pop or orange juice. Go without gluten, pasta, bread, potatoes and milk for a month to see how you feel without them. Buy green vegetables and fruit. No liquid drinks except water should be in your refrigerator. Buy a case of low sodium club soda for salt replacement if you are going to fast. Do not eat out to socialize as a habit. Fill yourself with pleasure in non-eating ways.

*Find snacks such as vegetables with high fiber and low sugar. Use decaffeinated products instead of caffeine. Use delay techniques before bad habits. Substitute and encourage creativity. Treats are not nice when they are candy and soda pop. Realize cookies were never healthy. Living is healthy.

*Restructure your kitchen, clean out your pantry and your refrigerator. Do you hide candy because you think of it as a reward? When you see chocolate or dessert, remind yourself it is not helping you.

*Use smaller bowls, smaller plates and narrow glasses to decrease the amount you consume.

*Commit to never eating fried or breaded foods again.

*Certain foods make us feel bad--and we actually become addicted to eating the foods that alter our energy in the ways they do. Make your favorite snack a healthy snack. It's not "sweet dreams" but healthy dreams that matter.

*When six hours go by like one, then you are involved with life and doing the right thing. You have to invent, reinvent, experiment and remember what you enjoy in life. Whatever happens, say "I am not stressed by that, everything will be alright." Remind yourself to laugh.

*If you tend to overeat always at the same time of day, then plan intentional countering activities at that time in advance. Remember, nothing tastes as good as the feeling of less weight.

*Walk every day or whenever you're bored--a great commitment revitalizer. Walk whenever you can instead of driving or substitute bicycling. Do dishes by hand and let the dishwasher rest.

*Tricks of the Trade: Trade health food for bad food. Trade fresh mineral water for any other liquid drink, especially sodas. Trade walking and exercise for boredom. Trade joy for stress, and peace for worry or anxiety–either through meditation or self-talk.

Modern life today is like someone sitting you in a chair, putting extreme pressures on you --then they offer you hot bread, sweet candy and chocolate to eat as relief. You've been doing the eating but realize you've also been doing most of the torture to yourself through your life choices.

The lips and face are represented much higher in the brain and have much more influence on sensation than much of the rest of the body. Therefore, sipping coffee from a cup, using your lips, biting and chewing all increase the sense of pleasure and/or stress relief. The goal is not to take away your pleasure from eating but reduce the time you needlessly eat, make it more healthy and pleasurable and give you *self-control over it rather than it controlling you.*

*Stop reflexive eating and being consumed with survival. *Give yourself a one-year goal.* Once you start on the path to losing weight, you can reinforce your habits by daily weighing for one month, then weekly and so on. Eventually, you need to not care about your daily weight as much as are you active and healthy. Take your physical goal, emotional goal, mental goal, exercise goal, eating goal, home goal and work goal to completion and make new ones to march you to success.

*Make time for yourself. Some people don't take time for themselves or express themselves. You've got to change that and take a selfish allotment of time for yourself to be in balance on earth. To maintain your body, emotions and mind you have to maintain health. **When you think of food, ask yourself this question: "Will this food help me or hurt me?"**

*Decide on a plan where you have a smaller meal when you don't exercise, but eat more when you do. This may work to motivate you to exercise when you might not otherwise get going. Seeing your physique in the mirror may motivate you. Reminding yourself that you want to be alive when your children/grandchildren are older may motivate you. Being able to do some activities you could enjoy may motivate you. You really need to take a look at your personal drives to determine what *you* need for motivation.

*Losing weight or maintaining an ideal healthy weight often

comes down to allowing happiness in your life. You need to find the head/heart habit of being happy and balanced. It may require you doing a few things differently. How you see yourself is important. Visualize your look, your leanness, your physical prowess, your capability, your mental elevation and your freedom to go anywhere.

*Nutrient dense, low carbohydrate, low fat, vegetarian, mostly raw foods using goat or sheep dairy products and the grains quinoa and amaranth will likely be optimum for most people. Rice, pasta and potatoes and meaty meals can be eaten optionally on days that you exercise more.

*The pros of losing weight are that you can cross your legs, live longer, be able to do more, go swimming, walk farther and smell better. You can have mirrors in the house, decrease your blood pressure, decrease the likelihood of diabetes, cure diabetes, cure hypertension, and wear more types of clothes. **Everyone who is overweight is on the road to having diabetes!** You may have it or metabolic syndrome now and not even know it. While your sugar levels may always check normal, your insulin levels may be going higher and higher as your insulin resistance goes up. The insulin levels retain sodium from the kidneys and you can begin to have high blood pressure before ever showing blood sugar changes. Only after passing these stages do you actually become diabetic with uncontrolled sugar levels. You may be at more risk than you think.

Other cons are illness, depression, difficulty in traveling, needing special chairs to sit in, sleep apnea, GERD, heart disease and the list goes on.

*If you don't like something about yourself, don't be sad. Start to do something by making the change. Educate yourself and begin to make changes one at a time. Consciously and unconsciously, a new internal programming will click and things will start to move and shift to manifest what is best within your psyche.

*Divide the day into increments. How you handle yourself during these times can be easier when you focus your goals for that time period. Consider the day from morning 8-12am, afternoon 12-3 and 3-6, then evening 6-12pm. Seeing the day pass in increments may help with time specific challenges to eat or exercise. Conquer each segment of the day by dividing it up into temptations to respond differently.

*Don't over-salt, over-butter or over-sugar your food preparation. Even a little weight loss significantly helps your health parameters. Your food plan may be to decrease meat consumption while maintaining appropriate protein. Use low-glycemic load vegetables and fruit. Plan and invest in one change at a time. Change one week at a time.

*You have to invest some educational time to find new foods and ways of preparation. You need to expand your food preparation choices for variety's sake. Buy an appealing raw food preparation book.

A key is to make raw food or any healthier vegetarian food good and fun with variety. Change holiday food rituals weeks in advance of the actual holiday so you don't revert to historical or cultural high fat, high carbohydrate foods. Substitute! Create a healthy home food environment. You need right foods, right thoughts, right activities and right emotions to be healthy. You can maintain yourself, one thought at time, one emotion at a time and one food at a time that you choose to eat or choose not to eat.

*The *Inside-Outside Diet* is about changing your inner you, mental you, emotions and how you function. Your body will change in response to the invisible blueprint of your inner life and become *permanent* when the new habits are strengthened.

You create you from the Inside-Out. You respond from the Outside-In. **Choices that we make, even when we think we're not choosing is a choice to continue as we are.** Knowledge, options and persistence make us complete. We resume our inheritance of emotionally, consciously living by our sustained awareness.

*Identify the challenges that could upset your meeting your goals. Use a bracelet to remind yourself about goals: e.g. lose 10 pounds, make a mental change, an emotional change, a lifestyle change or an exercise goal.

*Make a return visit to your doctor for guidance and check your health.

*Keep weekly visits with your therapist or doctor to maintain your motivations and solutions. Your money will be well spent on improving your health.

*Be patient with yourself. Your long-term commitment is to *eventually* be happier, but it probably won't happen without some struggle and relapses before the triumph.

*Maintaining an ideal weight is less rewarding than is the initial loss of weight. Dietary monotony can be relieved with new, healthy cookbook recipes. Exercise routines can be varied for stimulation and enthusiasm.

*You need a maintenance program: an individual plan of foods you can eat or not, a list of allergenic foods, the golden foods and supplements, behavioral support, lifestyle changes, emotional freedom, mental self awareness, and an exercise plan which you solidify and make regular.

*With obesity as an illness rising to number one in the population, you could socially, medically, and legally justify most junk food items being banned from advertising just as alcohol and tobacco ads were removed for the same reasons. I'd like a change at all grocery stores so they won't place all their addictive candy and soda pop junk food at the impulse buying check-out lanes.

*For growing children and young adults, let the kids grow out of the weight, and don't panic. Try to get the schools to take the candy and soda pop vending machines out of the schools. Don't stress them about being overweight and force them on a weight-loss diet. Normalize food habits, their social environment and allow time for good health to replace poor health. Children need parental participation to lose weight so parenting skills and your example are important.

*Life isn't static. What will work for you now as motivation and maintenance may not work for you in three-to-six months. So recheck and reset your goals every two months until you achieve your healthy weight goal. You may need to do more, do something different than you did in the beginning or reread this very book for more examples you can do. Refine your food choices more, expand and explore for variety.

*Know yourself well. Denial just puts off self knowledge, and, in terms of learning to manage your weight, gets you nowhere. Momentary indulges can be forgiven, but understand why you lapsed, how frequently, and what you could have done instead. Take this example:

I had a patient, who I'll call Sally, who maintained 95 percent of her day with great determination. She worked an upper level job at a big company. Sally was overweight about 30 pounds and had a body fat of 28 percent. She ate well 95 percent of the time and she even exercised two times a week, though her work outs were not that strenuous and short in quality. She was very even tempered and in perhaps too much control of her emotions. Then about once a week, Sally would binge on chocolate and soft drinks, not sleep and feel terrible the next day. Part of her not feeling well the next day would have been appropriate due to the "drugs" she consumed the night before. Part of her not feeling well the next day was unnecessary because she was getting down on herself because of the "failure."

First, Sally needed to know she should not condemn herself for getting ahead and then having a setback. She needed to see herself and her actions as a series of factors causing her to act as she did. We focused on the causation.

Sally accepted that she was making the decisions. She realized that she still had elements of negative self-esteem that she was burdened with when she failed--with imprinted emotional elements of this going back all through high school. Sally knew she had to help herself and started with positive affirmations about herself to affirm her worth. She also realized that she intellectually got the picture of what she was doing with herself but she had not *emotionally* gotten the reality of what she was doing in her life. She was controlling too much of her emotional stream of energy with work, husband and children. She never really relaxed and she was still a bit too driven for her own good and ability to exercise happily.

The emotional exercises Sally did had to be repeated more frequently and she needed to let her hair down a little more often. She also needed to talk with her children and husband for their understanding of what she was doing. Not being overweight, they never really understood her motivations and what she was doing to improve her life. When she eventually "got it" at a deeper level in her heart, she understood what emotional freedom was. It was not just an intellectual concept but a concept to live by.

Finally, Sally started to accomplish her goal of reaching an ideal health and weight. She did not just suddenly stop binging on chocolate and soda, but she used it less frequently until she was able to stop completely. She accomplished for herself something long lasting and built her own empowerment. I have no doubt that with even more time she will continue the direction of total self mastery.

Everything bad for you that you don't eat puts you on the road to recovery. Every time you say no, you get more. Make a plan and practice walking through it. If you just write it down it doesn't have mental memory or emotional memory. You must apply and practice the steps to achieve them.

You might have hundreds of memory experiences of eating a chocolate ice cream sundae and saying it felt good even if it really made you feel bad, and it added on pounds and made you depressed later on.

What it meant to you, which is an ingrained pattern now, will come out again as a solution when you feel, say stress. You can self-talk and enact new patterns but they require many repetitions to become dominant. Don't worry if you fall off the wagon and eat old foods. It is normal and a way of learning. The frequency becomes less and less with mental restructuring and re-labeling of your conscious choices. Don't get down on yourself for occasional relapses, you will change at your pace and learn from the repetitions.

Ayurvedically speaking, with this high stress world, most vata lowering or stress-lowering foods happen to be kapha increasing which means weight increasing. "The Golden Foods" are those foods that decrease vata (stress) and kapha (body mass). *Perfect peace tea* balances all three doshas and the Golden Food list helps balance the primary vata stress and overweight kapha tendencies.

The reason this culture has increased problems is the combination of stress, boredom and a huge supply of food items, some very unhealthy. Increased availability and financial ability to buy food is everywhere. People have the ability to stay at home, do little, work little and eat a lot. Survival doesn't require activity for most people now. You don't even have to get up to turn the television on anymore. Financial survival and materialism are false drives burdening the modern day societies adding unnecessary stress to people's lives. Food manufacturer's commercials are constantly trying to tell you their food will bring "meaning" to your life – it never will, it is a deceitful if not malignant manipulation.

Before you start, ask yourself, "How much are you willing to alter your life?" How ready are you to alter things, the way you live, your job, how you think and the food that you buy? Are you willing to read a recipe book and will you make the time for these necessary things in your life that are required to be different? This is a very important gauge for you to know how well you are prepared to succeed.

The *Inside-Outside* changes are meant to work long term.

Implement them over time. After all, how long has it taken you to become overweight or overfat? You must be patient for the changes you want to make to become secure in your psyche, but knowing this, you also must start! Do what you can do, think only of succeeding and toss everything else that held you back in the past.

Let me summarize further the main points for you here:

*Read, educate yourself and become aware.

*Implement what's most important to you of what you read.

*Discontinue mind-affecting foods, drinks and addictive foods and drinks. Allow a two week withdrawal period. Expect it.

*Take high quality vitamin supplements and amino acid supplements for the weight loss period.

*Start walking. For exercise setbacks, motivate yourself! On a piece of paper, list the benefits of exercise, strength training and walking versus continuing as you are. For example, you gain energy and strength rather than continue feeling sluggish and out of shape. Reviewing this comparison list will inspire you to rethink what you want out of life. The simple truth is that you need to retrain your mind to alter self-sabotaging habits.

*Start evaluating your 24 hour routine by time of day.

*Keep on noticing your habits of when you feel stress or overwhelming boredom.

*Start becoming aware of your mind set and emotional responses. Do you eat for pleasure, boredom or relief from stress and anxiety?

*Consider a change of job.

*If you have deeper unresolved problem drives, work with a psychologist or hypnotherapist or try evaluating and correcting yourself.

*Fasting is an option that is natural and very powerful. Start off slowly.

*Start increasing your physical activity by making time for it in your week.

*Which of these four mechanisms of overeating or becoming "over fat" do you partake in: a) overeating for stress relief, b) overeating for pleasure, c) not exercising due to having no time. (stress), d) not exercising due to a very negative imprinted attitude about working out or your body? Know yourself! Don't distort the truth.

*If you don't have enthusiasm for life then you are ruled by fears—and you must know why.

*Remind yourself that eating is often equal to avoiding facing threats. Learn to confront fears and threats or overeating will be the result.

*An over-commitment to materialism increases stress.

*Too many internal conflicts? Simplify your life. Stop being frustrated, take your time and give yourself reasonable daily goals and days with no goals whatsoever. Accomplish only one goal each day.

*Use non-eating ways to increase pleasure and dump stress.

Finally, when you are caught off guard and your personal demon demands that you take the lid off the cookie jar for a reward, stop yourself! Take a deep breath and figure out if you are feeling over-stressed or under-satisfied. Confront the truth and self-talk yourself through the automatic mindless cookie moments to something more important: the reality of your good health.

*Next, by recognizing your blocks to making physical activity a routine aspect of your life, you work with the *Inside-Outside* techniques of change. As a helpmate, both a daily plan and weekly plan of physical activity will regulate your improvements.

*Once you learn how to make these techniques your own, you will be able to tune into them to keep you ever healthy--inside and out. You will have vastly increased your knowledge of your health and that knowledge will endow you with everlasting power and fulfilling life.

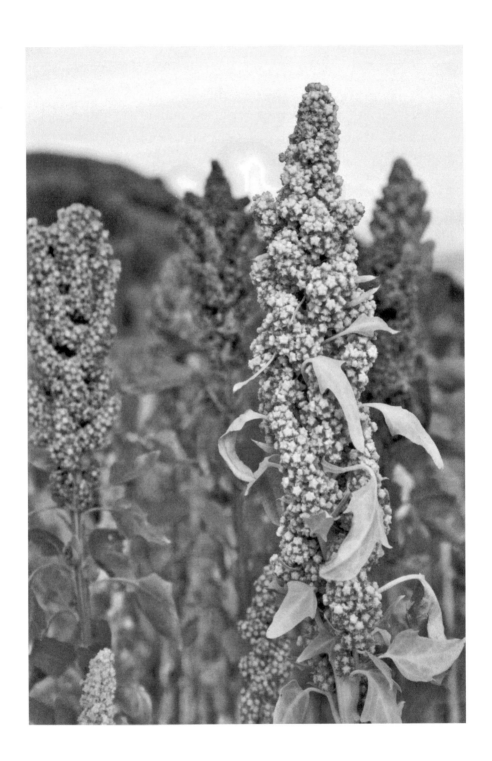

Appendix
Guides, Tools and Therapy

The Golden Foods

To start you out, here's a comprehensive list of <u>The Golden Foods</u>, foods that both decrease stress and weight according to ayurveda. The foods to be sure to *avoid* are listed on the right side.

Foods that tend to stabilize stress and weight. (Decrease kapha, vata, and neutral pitta)

FOODS best to USE: **FOODS NOT to Consume**:

Fruits:

Apricots, berries, cherries, mango-ripe, peaches, soaked raisins, strawberries, some grapes, kiwi, lemons, limes

watermelon, dried fruit, frozen fruit, fruit with sugar,

Vegetables:

Artichoke, asparagus, bean sprouts, beets, daikon radish, fenugreek greens, cooked garlic, well-cooked green beans, horseradish, cooked leeks, mache, cooked okra, cooked onions, **RADISH**, scallopini squash, cooked shallots,

pickled vegetables, tomatoes, spaghetti squash

summer squash, watercress, **RED BEETS**
crooked-neck yellow squash, zucchini,
SWEET CARROTS

Grains:

Amaranth, cooked oats, basmati rice,   cold cereal
wheat bran

Animal Foods:

Poached eggs, some chicken or turkey   beef, lamb, pork, venison

Legumes:

Soaked and well-cooked legumes,   kidney beans,
adzuki beans, **RED LENTILS**,   soy flour, soy powder,
tepary beans, hot tofu, tur dal   tempeh, common lentils,
                            soy margarine, soy beans,

Nuts:

Almonds -well-soaked   peanuts

Seeds:

Chia, flax, sunflower, pumpkin   psyllium

Sweeteners:

Fruit juice concentrates esp. apple, pear   white sugar

Condiments:

Black pepper, coriander leaves,   ketchup
daikon radish, garlic, ghee, fresh ginger,
horseradish, lettuce, mint leaves, mustard,
cooked onions, radishes

Spices

Ajwan, allspice, anise, asafetida, basil,   almond extract, tamarind,
bay leaf, black pepper, caraway,   neem leaves, amchoor
cayenne, cinnamon, cloves, coriander,
cumin, dill, fennel, fenugreek, garlic,
ginger, horseradish, mace, marjoram, mint,
mustard seeds, cooked onion, orange peel,
oregano, paprika, parsley, peppermint,
pippali, poppy seeds, rosemary, rose water,
saffron, sage, savory, spearmint, star anise,
tarragon, thyme, turmeric, vanilla,
wintergreen, **ANISE SEEDS**
CARDAMON, CELERY SEED

Dairy:

Ghee, freshly made yogurt,   all not fresh dairy,
fresh goat's milk   ice cream, sour cream,
                                                    hard cheeses, cow's milk

Oils:

Cold fresh-pressed oils, **SAFFLOWER OIL, WHITE MUSTARD OIL**	deep-fried or rancid oils,

Beverages:

Aloe vera juice, apricot juice, berry juice, carrot juice, carrot-ginger juice, hot-spiced goat milk, cherry juice, grape juice, mango juice, peach nectar, low-salt vegetable bouillons	carbonated drinks, icy cold drinks, alcohol, grain beverages, cold dairy products, tomato juice, V-8 juice,

Teas:

Ajwan, basil, catnip, chamomile, cinnamon, cloves, ginseng, hawthorne, juniper berries, lavender, lemon balm, lemon grass, orange peel, osha, pennyroyal, peppermint, raspberry, rose flowers, saffron, sage, sarsaparilla, sassafras, wild ginger

Others:

Spirulina, blue-green algae	chlorella

Here's the <u>progress and goal charts</u> that I refer to in my office. Though they always have to be individualized, they provide structure that helps promote weight loss success. They are filled with goals and simple strategies that need to be implemented. Emotional frustrations, as a common element of anyone's life who is already overweight must be anticipated, expected and planned. Keep weekly doctor visits for the first two months to strengthen your motivation and the small triumphs you enact in your life.

I have found in practice that giving anyone more than eight tasks to complete in terms of changing habits is too much. Sometimes, one task must be focused on alone to achieve it. So I use these plans that are accomplished over as long as necessary. I do not go on until I know everything in phase one is being undertaken or has been accomplished. With these plans, individuality must always be considered and can modify the plans for anyone's special health concerns. It is important to elevate the peace and pleasure states of people before directly taking on their hidden mental resistance.

Plan & Commitment to Change

The goal in the first week is to develop food knowledge, supplement for critical nutrient deficiencies, and read all food labels to remove foreign food from your intake. Most supplements given will only be taken for 30 to 60 days and then not used after that.

First Actions & Goals:

A   Stop all Unnatural Foods.
ACTION - Implement reading all food labels, understand what the labels mean.

B   Supplement for overall health. Replenishing all essential nutrient elements for body health - vitamins, minerals, co-factors, omega 3 and 6 fatty acids.
ACTION - Take high quality basic nutrients, trace minerals, chromium, vanadium, calcium/magnesium and essential fatty acids. Stop all other supplements you are taking.

C   Physical ASSESSMENT
ACTION - Measure your % Body Fat, Overall Weight & Waist circumference. Start simple 5 minute morning stretching warm-up.

D   Emotional Self-Observation
ACTION - Begin to observe yourself & Become AWARE of WHY you eat & HOW you feel before the urge to eat. These are self-notes as to "WHY YOU EAT WHEN YOU DO."

E   Food Nutrient Correction
ACTION - Stop all breads, pastas, potatoes, cereals, gluten grains, liquid drinks (other than mineralized water) sugar, desserts & cow dairy products. You can use ghee as a substitute

for butter. You can use goat yogurt, sheep yogurt, goat cheese or sheep cheeses. Experiment for the ones you like. You can eat all the non-citrus fruit and vegetables you like, preferred more raw types of eating. Meat is okay for now if you like but vegetarian is a goal. This is done for partly therapeutic reasons and partly as a test to see if cravings develop.

F   SELF-EDUCATION

ACTION - Must READ book, *Start Living, Stop Dying – 10 Steps to Natural Health by* Mark E Laursen MD, NMD, ABHM as your foundation to natural health.

G   Health & Laboratory Analysis

ACTION - Specific labs ordered for you which will include as a basis Chem 24 with lipids, Complete Blood Count with differential (CBC), TSH, T-4, free T-3 thyroid testing, Hemoglobin A1-c, 10-part Urinalysis, Pulse oximetry. Optional tests are: C reactive protein, insulin levels, Blood type (if not known). Individual labs or procedures may be ordered for your individual health history and current condition.

H   Admonition for PATIENCE. The goal is to think of one year for permanence.

ACTION - Please be advised a complete restructuring of your foundation is underway and that you will need the development of total patience for this program of replenishment and revitalization.

A complete holistic health history and physical examination will be completed prior to starting the program.

Second Actions & Goals:

The second period is to increase knowledge, supplement for sleep and stress. Treat any neurohormonal imbalance or anxiety reactions with amino acids. Treat any cravings or addictions with amino acids initially. Continue stretching and START exercising. Discuss good food.

You must treat individual health problems along the way. During the second phase, use supplements, expand exercise program, re-evaluate lifestyle. Each week, discuss your emotional goal, physical goal, mental goal and life goal. Individual therapy as necessary.

A   Follow-up of unnatural foods. Are you understanding food ingredients and why this is important to improve?
ACTION - Home pantry Clean-up. Task is to go through your pantry and throw away ALL your foods that have unnatural ingredients in them. IT IS BETTER FOR UNNATURAL FOODS TO GO TO WASTE THAN TO GO TO YOUR WAIST!
ACTION - As you go to the grocery store, you initially have to spend more time looking at the food labels of all the manufacturers of food, to see who makes the best natural product for the type of food you are willing to buy. In some cases you cannot buy any of the product type that you planned. Raw and/or organic foods will be better. Use more fruits and vegetables in your menu.
B   Follow-up of nutritional supplements. How are supplements going and how do you feel.
ACTION - Adjust supplements according to individual.
C   Supplement for Weight Loss & Natural Detoxification & Individual Concerns & Needs.

ACTION - Take natural vitamin E mixed tocopherols, selenium, Vitamin C with flavanoids, zinc picolinate, Tyrosine with iodine for thyroid function & carnityl. As you lose WEIGHT, you will naturally lose the fat-bound toxins and poisons (PCB's and heavy metals) that tend to accumulate & are bound in fat cells. You need early protection from these released chemicals.

D   Observation for types of foods that constitute cravings or addictions and snack foods.

ACTION - Take written notes in a **7 day journal** of what types of snacks or foods you crave or have as an addiction. Note HOW YOU FEEL in a journal when you eat or want to eat these foods. Show this journal at our visit. Relate eating drives to your energy states.

E   Decrease food portions and volume.

ACTION - DRINK (1) 8 oz glass of water prior to all eating of snacks and meals.

ACTION - Restaurant eating (if you do). Bring half of food ordered home so you eat half as much as what is served. You will have an extra meal at home to eat later. You quit eating earlier in a meal leaving food on your plate. You will notice you do become satisfied shortly after stopping eating and you will be subconsciously saying, "I don't need anymore." as you do this.

F   Exercise

ACTION - START Walking. Best to do this first thing in morning and again at night. This will naturally motivate you, stimulating your bowels to empty & open you up to NATURE & pleasure in the daytime, & naturally de-stress you at night. If you can't walk, then a substitute exercise or activity must be implemented. Use home based exercise.

G   Follow-up on weight & waist circumference

        ACTION - Measure weight & waist circumference.

        Review all laboratory testing results on an individual basis.

        ACTION - Meet with your doctor to review results and any further plans or testing that may be needed as follow-up to your individual needs and health determinates. Dispense urine monitoring strips.

H   Implement raw, natural, organic salads, greens, steamed vegetables, stir fries and fruits. An optional Food replacement program may be continued for 2-4 weeks if already using. Action - Experiment with better natural foods. Optionally use Optifast, Nutrisystem, Weight-Watchers, Nutra-slim, Medifast, Metagenics, Jenny Craig etc. Keep in mind you MUST begin to gain knowledge of natural foods, that you will prepare naturally & eventually for best health & control.

Third Actions & Goals:

Goals are to increase physical activity, deepen the understanding of the food/emotional reaction pattern of your habits and understanding how your mind works. Counter any resistance coming up in the mind. Optional fasting: one day fasts times three, and then a three-day fast to see how your body reacts. Personal blocks and habits may appear.

A   Prescription medication reduction of dose or elimination, when safely possible and when natural improvements make elimination of prescription drugs necessary.

        ACTION - Consultation to review which prescription drugs (if you take any) may be candidates for replacement or reduction. This is an individualized program of HEALTH.

B   Follow-up on UNNATURAL food elimination. How are you

doing with finding food replacements for your lifestyle and meals? Nuts and seeds provide protein if vegetarian.

ACTION - REFRIGERATOR CLEAN-UP. Go through your refrigerator and throw away any unnatural foods that are still present in your refrigerator. Read all their food labels. Find substitutes for any of these foods that you have not yet replaced with natural products.

C   Cravings and Food Addiction Follow-Up. Review your journal about any particular foods that are used for emotional substitutes, cravings and addictions. This is an individualized approach that you may not need.

ACTION - Supplement amino acid therapy for food addictions, cravings & overeating. This is a fatigue & anxiety amino acid supplement therapy. Use GABA, 5-HTP, d-phenylalanine, l-glutamine & theanine therapy as part of an individualized therapy. This is a therapy for specific emotional pattern eating.

D   Supplement follow-up. How do you feel with supplements. Most supplements are temporary. Continued behavioral therapy. Identifying origins of habits and beliefs.

ACTION - Thyroid supplementation continued. Add specific thyroid nutrients to iodine & tyrosine to contribute to proper thyroid functioning.

E   Overeating Analysis of WHY you overeat. Type of overeating: Boredom for PLEASURE, or STRESS/ANXIETY eating for relief, or combination.

ACTION - Review journal & personal notes of snack eating to determine what type of overeating person you have been.

F   EMOTIONAL THERAPY – Use the emotional healing exercises to heal. This is an individualized form of therapy. Some emotional exercises demonstrated.

ACTION - Increase pleasure exercise or stress release therapy.

G   Sleep evaluation. You must receive a good night's rest.

ACTION - Office evaluation for criteria that relate to sleeping easily.

Use limited water intake at night and drinking water in the morning. Thought-extinguishing exercise if needed.

Fourth Actions & Goals:

Goals are to develop reinforcement and maintenance program to allow independent monitoring of your program. Continue any personal therapy reinforcement. Exercise to use "powerplate technology" (vibrational strength training/metabolic rate stimulation) or resistance therapy/exercise. Remember, habits will return and backsliding is normal and is not a sign of failure. Reset Goals.

A   Food intake follow-up.
        ACTION - Review Food shopping, Only purchase food after
        having eaten & dinner. Always buy food using a list and
        MUST always shop for food after having recently finished a
        meal. Elimination of food shopping while potentially hungry.
        AWARENESS of Impulse food displays by food stores and
        other business establishments that do not concern themselves
        with your health.
B   Constipation & Detoxification. People with a long history
        of constipation and toxin exposure or with known toxicity
        organ overload problems (skin problems, lung problems, liver
        problems, kidney problems or bowel problems) should concern
        themselves with whether a colonic cleanse followed by a
        probiotic re-colonization would be therapeutic.
        ACTION - Consider a COLON CLEANSE consultation and
therapy.

C   EDUCATION. Nutrition, health and diet.
        ACTION - Read *The Inside-Outside Diet – Lose the Emotional weight, Lose the Mental Weight, Lose the Physical Weight* by Mark E. Laursen MD, NMD, ABHM.

D   Physical Assessment – Measure weight, BMI, waist circumference, specific body diameter, % body fat.
        ACTION - Office visit to measure the above parameters of health.

E   Exercise follow-up
        ACTION - Implement scheduled walking, plan time of day. Plan lean muscle mass gaining. Review mental causes for decreased willpower to go ahead with exercise.

F   Mental - Emotional therapy. These personal and individualized therapies may need to be additionally scheduled for your needs, obstacles and goals.
        ACTION - Individualized behavioral therapy for your stress or pleasure based re-correction of eating. Substitute.

G   Fasting Therapy
        ACTION - Implement fasts per individual desire, self-analysis, and development of self-monitoring.

The use of individual therapy and guided exercises continues here and is dependent upon the individual involved in terms of what they need as the core of their success. How much *Inside* work you have to do is variable among different people. How deep you have to know yourself to create change is also variable because for some people they only have a limited mental-emotional obstacle that has been driving them to overeat. For some, once they "see" it, they get it. For other people, there are layers of emotions and beliefs that they must peel off one by one to improve to the next level. However, each improvement does bring them closer to empowerment and a better weight.

We also realize that *telling* how one's inner reality works is one thing and demonstrating how to *do* something is another. Like any course work, some people get it quicker than others, yet everyone can get it. With food, supplements, herbs and even exercise you can touch it, feel it, identify these things and then control it. With emotions, thoughts and drives the first step is to become aware of them and *identify them.* To begin, you identify which emotional energies you are experiencing with overeating: stress energy, or boredom and pleasure or both combined. Second, identify the environment you are responding to when you feel overeating energies inside you.

When you are feeling an uncomfortable need for pleasure drives, what are the circumstances? Are you allowing yourself to interact in the world to bring that joyful interaction to you from the environment? You can allow yourself to feel more by becoming aware that you are limiting your emotions, then use the emotional expansion and freedom exercises to re-expand your sensual awareness and enjoyment.

For stress you follow a different inward algorithm. It still starts with identifying environment triggers that build the stress within you. These triggers can be other people that conflict with you or your very own beliefs that are too ridiculous to get along in the world peacefully. If the stress is from other people you need to ask why you go along with it–you don't have to join the crowd of irritation all around you. Remember who you are and what choices you are making.

Within yourself you need to ask yourself what beliefs in your very own mind create the worry and stress within you. You will have other beliefs that lead you into conflict and survival thinking that must be contemplated and understood and released. Can you simplify?

Classification of Therapy by Naturalness

Tier 0

Thoughts, beliefs;
Emotions, feeling;
Contemplation
Meditation
Visualization

Tier 1

Food elimination
Food intentional eating
Lifestyle – Body Changes
Feng shui changes
Environmental Changes

Tier 2

Supplements – Natural
Minerals, trace minerals
Vitamins & co-factors
Essential Fatty acids

Tier 3

Herbal remedies
Chinese herbs
Ayurvedic herbs
American/Native herbs

Tier 4

Prescription Medication – Synthetic
Chemotherapy

Tier 5

Surgery – any kind.
Radiation

Supplement Therapy:

All the supplements I use are from a few high quality manufacturers. Use these OTC nutrients only with the advice of a professional.

Phases of Supplement Therapies:

Phase I - Basic Health Nutrients

Basic vitamins, minerals & co-factors, trace minerals and omega 3 essential fatty acids.

These are the basic nutrients I would suggest for anyone for average life conditions.

Phase II - Natural Anti-Oxidant Nutrients

Selenium, zinc, vitamin C and natural vitamin E.

These make up the core of your most natural anti-cancer, anti-free radical cellular protection in your body. Because fat can store and release toxins, these nutrients are important to supplement while losing weight.

Phase III - Weight-Loss Nutrients

Carnitine, chromium, vanadium, Co Q 10, iodine, tyrosine and thyroid nutrients.

These are the natural nutrients specifically needed by your body for fat and sugar metabolism and for your thyroid to function properly.

Phase IV - Neurohormonal Nutrients

Optional amino acid therapy for cravings and addictions or sleep disturbances.

Glutamine, 5-HTP, d-phenylalanine, GABA, l-tyrosine.

www.NaturalBodyHealth.com

The 7-7-7 Plan to Rapid Health

This is a do-it-yourself weekly approach to gradually but quickly, transition to a healthier food plan and activity level. The plan starts by you going to the grocery store and buying all the vegetables and fruit you like. Buy hard apples and soft bananas for your home. For this first week, you will eat all the vegetables for meals you like and all the fruit for snacks and dessert that you like. Buy at least one new fruit or vegetable each grocery store visit so that you can try one new food each week. Take all the meat from your refrigerator and feed it to the dogs or give it away or throw it away. You will have no meat for this week. On day 3, go to the store again and replenish your vegetables and fruit but go only after you have eaten lunch or dinner.

Starting this first week, I want you to say nothing negative or of a conflict nature to anyone. Nor do you even think of anything negative about anything or anyone *and this includes yourself.* You have to do this for an entire week. If you forget, then you have to start over again and go for another week. You will notice how often you put yourself down or others down and notice how this drops your energy to a lower level. This will force you to keep your positive energy up and out. If you catch yourself thinking anything contradictory you must rethink it or say it in an encouraging hopeful manner. This will greatly affect your energy for the day and keep many of the harmful energy changes from occurring.

The next 7 days you go to the health food store and buy 6 or 32 oz of goat yogurt and 2 kinds of sheep or goat cheese. I suggest you buy "mancheca" goat cheese as it tastes very similar to cow cheese. As an option you can buy goat milk but you can also buy almond milk or rice milk to substitute for cow milk. Buy cold expeller pressed sunflower oil to be used in any non-cooking food preparations. Buy cold expeller pressed virgin olive oil to be used for any cooking or stir fry. As an option you can purchase safflower oil or coconut oil for cooking. You can also buy walnut oil, grapeseed oil or sesame oil if this fits your type of cooking/food preparation desires. From your refrigerator take all the cow milk and cow cheeses, and give them to your dogs or throw them away. You will now have gone "cow dairy free. "

Carry the fruit and vegetables forward and your "positive expressions" to this week so you are still non-meat and non-negativity. Try a new sheep or goat cheese each week and keep a written list of all the ones you have liked so you can remember to buy them again in the future.

The third week you will go to the health food store and buy the grain quinoa. Use quinoa at home as a substitute for rice. Take all your breads, pancake mixes and cereals and throw them out or give them away to those less fortunate and if they take them they will indeed be less fortunate. Throw away all your oats and barley also. Cook quinoa like rice and eat it with meals hot, or let it cool and keep it in your refrigerator to use it cold with salads. You will now be gluten free. As an option, you can purchase amaranth, buckwheat or millet as they are also gluten free. Using these 3 non-gluten foods will expand your variety and will require some experimentation with alternative recipes of food preparation.

Carry all your non-meat, non-cow dairy and pro-positivity forward to this week.

The 4th week you've gone this far, why not go all the way forward. Stop all coffee, black tea, green tea, msg chip products, chocolate, soda pop, candy, nicotine and alcohol. With this bold move you will stop all the mood destroying products that have been manipulating your psyche up and down and all around. Carry all of this forward. Fruit will be your snacks and dessert. Vegetables in all variety will be your food entertainment. New foods like amaranth, quinoa and millet will be your creativity. Life will be for the first time since you were 2 years old, fresh and positive as it is supposed to be again.

You will now have accomplished a vegetarian, cow dairy free, gluten free, anti-diabetes, anti-arthritis, anti-autism, anti-depression, mood stabilizing food program that will be 95% right for your body. The remaining 5% is because you might have individual food allergens that you shouldn't eat and you will need to eat seasonally to have the remaining 100% accomplished. You will have the food program that may reverse atherosclerosis in your body.

Now we'll add your body to the program.

On day one of the next week, get up in the morning and go sit on the floor. Take one foot at a time and rotate your foot around in both directions to fully wake up your ankles with this range of motion exercise. Next, slide your hands up your legs to your hips.

Sit on the floor with one leg forward and the other bent back at the knee known as a "hurdle" stretch. Lean forward and hold it for 30 seconds to stretch your hamstring muscles. Do each leg. Now sit on the floor with your legs apart in the "splits." It doesn't matter how far apart you have your legs for now. Lean to the right, then forward and then left. Repeat each hold for 30 seconds again.

Now place your feet flat on the floor as if you are about to stand up but sit with your knees bent in this crouched position. Slowly straighten your knees as you raise your hips up but keep your head down so that you are in a "jack-knife" position. Place your hands on the floor or as far down to the floor as they will go. Slowly, slowly, one vertebrae at a time, begin to roll your back up starting with your sacrum and go all the way to your neck to elevate your head to a normal position. Roll your head to the left a full circle and then to the right slowly. Bend your head to the left and then to the right. Turn your head to the left and then to the right. Rotate your arms around like a windmill slowly front and then back in a complete circle, left and right arms. Now find a wall to lean forward keeping your heels on the floor to stretch your calves and hamstrings again. You are done with the stretch. This takes 5 to 10 minutes is all. Do this stretch 3 times a week

Now go sit in front of an east facing window where the sun comes up and sit on the floor and look in the direction of the sun for 10 minutes. Close your eyes if the sun is too bright or look in the general direction of the sun. If the sun is first coming up you can probably look directly at it for this time. Do this morning sun sitting 3 times a week. The sun acts as an energy catalyst forming vitamin D3 in your skin and stimulating health, and the sun counters depressive moods on a neurohormonal basis.

The second week, carry everything forward. Buy a jump rope. In the morning after you stretch do 3 sets of 12 sit-ups rolling forward, push-ups, jumping jacks, "burpees" and jump rope. You set the number you want to do. Do these calisthenics 3 times a week.

The third week add walking to your plan. This can be done anytime of day, preferably in nature and be observant of your surroundings as you walk. Walk to the distance you can easily accomplish and slowly lengthen the time or distance or frequency you walk.

You will now have put your body in motion that will generate more good moods, detoxification and global healing of your life.

If you have not gotten to the end of this quick induction to health and you have not simplified your life, then your lack of pleasure will return you to eating for pleasure once again. If you haven't become patient enough by this time, then the stress of your work will overwhelm you with overeating impulses once again. If you haven't increased your allowance of positivity into your life then your time for exercise will give way to what your consciousness tells you to do to survive - and you'll be back where you started, almost.

The Inside-Outside Review – For Patients

We start out, partially as a test and partly as a therapeutic practice, asking you to eat all the natural nutrient dense foods available which are mostly vegetables and fruit. No pasta, breaded foods and no starchy foods like white potatoes or bread. This is a modified vegetarian Paleolithic food plan that eliminates the common digestive difficulty foods such as cow dairy and gluten. Foods include the Golden Foods such as nuts, seeds, poached eggs, vegetables, fruit, quinoa and amaranth grains, mineralized water and some teas. Eliminating all cow dairy and gluten may be the most important food changes people can make to cure their ills.

We ask you to avoid all foods that affect mood and weaken the internal willpower. That means no caffeine (chocolate, coffee, green or black teas), msg or "sugar" products. We ask everyone who might smoke to stop or start to cut back to eliminate nicotine effects. Most people who start already do not smoke.

The only liquid drink you can have is mineralized water (not distilled like most bottled waters) or herbal teas. No juice drinks. No pastries or typical sugary desserts. No alcohol as it is a mood destabilizer.

We ask you to not have any unnatural food or allergenic foods. This means reading the food labels of everything bought or used, to eliminate unnatural ingredients. This effectively removes restaurant eating for the time being as you have no control or idea as to the ingredients when you don't prepare the food. No cow dairy or gluten (bread or cereal) or any food you know that individually gives you incompatible food symptoms or food allergy symptoms. No fast food establishments.

You can have meat if you like, but we ask you to choose to the left of a sliding scale of vegetarian, fish, fowl, lamb, pork and then beef foods. This means a primarily vegetarian food guide with natural raw being the more desirable, but not everyone can go into a raw food regimen immediately. Eating meat lends itself to more mood alterations so we choose away from it when deciding what to eat, yet we tell someone, "If you really have a drive to eat meat–go ahead and eat it for now."

At the same time, we supplement with the essential nutrients the body is required to consume from a very high quality supplement manufacturer. We do this to make up for any past or current deficiency of required nutrients. That is a multi-vitamin, co-factor and mineral supplement, calcium, magnesium, trace minerals and the two essential fatty acids: omega 3 and omega 6. By providing the body what it nutritionally needs from supplements and nutritionally dense foods, we eliminate the physical drives of the body for overeating. Often these supplements improve mood, satiety and thereby willpower.

By eliminating the "mood foods" we stabilize the emotions to allow for more willpower and clarity–essential for the *Inside-Out* powers to work. Those on caffeine and sugar drinks may feel headaches or withdrawal symptoms for one week before stabilizing.

We ask everyone to intentionally drink more water each day but to not drink after 7 or 8 p.m. (7 p.m. if you go to bed before 10 p.m. and no water after 8 p.m. if you go to bed after 10 p.m.) but drink a large glass of water first thing in the morning to keep with a "natural" lifestyle.

We do not advise to eat in the morning until you first begin to feel true hunger which usually would be between 9 and 11 a.m. We also want you to eat when you first notice feeling hungry and not put off eating until you are famished, otherwise your control for food selection and quantity will be diminished.

By doing these things we return everyone to a natural lifestyle relative to food and drink.

For breakfast you can have bananas, apples and eggs, yogurt (goat) and fruit like blueberries. For lunch you can have vegetables and quinoa or occasionally amaranth. Also, you can have some rice and fruit. Snacks can be any vegetable or non-citrus fruit. Nuts like Brazil nuts (never peanuts) can have appetite suppressing effect for some people due to their fat and protein content. Dinner (before 6 p.m.) can be fruit, nuts, seeds, quinoa, vegetables and spices.

Learn to substitute: cow milk for almond milk or rice milk

Grain - use quinoa, amaranth or occasional rice or millet.

Always have apples and bananas in house. Keep blueberries or blackberries in the refrigerator and other fruit as available. Stock up on goat and sheep cheeses and yogurts. Use vegetables as seasonally available.

We then ask everyone to keep track of the feelings they have prior to wanting to eat. Is it stress relief, boredom and a need for pleasure or true hunger? Start becoming aware. By tuning in to your feelings, we see if any particular food craving or addiction comes forward to present itself. If this happens we treat that specific individualized craving with the right amino acid therapy for four to eight weeks, we address emotional needs fulfilled by that craving and we address the original cause of that craving.

If you notice eating drives which are for pleasure or stress then we ask you to satisfy these emotional needs with non-eating methods. Start to look for the mental origins of these emotional drives.

Because many toxins are stored in fat tissue and will be released during fat loss, we do a secondary round of anti-oxidant, anti-cancer nutrient supplementation using natural mixed tocopherols (vitamin E), vitamin C, selenium and zinc. These provide safety in losing fat or fasting.

We ask you to take the time to add the three basic elements of exercise which are stretching, (I give a basic five-minute stretch); heart-lung aerobic activity such as walking, treadmill, bicycling, swimming or running; and we like some strength/resistance training to build some muscle mass and increase the resting metabolic rate. We may use "powerplate" vibration technology for muscle activity and exercise for those who cannot move as easily due to weight or joint limitations. We want to try and start an abdominal toning exercise such as jumping rope, running or trampoline methods that provide an up/down gravity motion to provide natural tone to the abdomen with activity.

We ask you to go cool with bathing or intentional cooling hydrotherapy to increase the basal metabolic rate. Strength training also increases the basal metabolic rate.

We try to individually reduce or eliminate excessive herbal and prescription drug usage that may be weakening you or causing too heavy a burden of toxicity. We attempt some early detoxification depending upon the individual. Steaming no more than once a week helps purify the body and detoxify the skin. The natural food regimen automatically helps the bowel function and detoxification but we may ask you in the second or third month to have bowel cleaning and sweeping therapy using specific herbs and/or hydrotherapy. Later, liver or blood cleansing may be provided.

We do check weight and percent body fat at intervals along the way for motivation and guidance.

All the while we emphasize the real internal emotional and mental you to become more aware of itself which it naturally will want to do. Specifically assigned emotional exercises are given to free and balance the human spirit. These are key. Personal aspects of mood or depression are addressed and individualization of the process occurs. Food choices, food compatibilities, prescription medication and exercise choices or limits are all addressed.

We advise patience and a long term perspective to weight loss and the regaining of a healthy life. We realize it takes many months to one year to replace 300 or so short term memory experiences that will want to remind you of what you have done to handle certain emotional situations like stress or lack of pleasure. It takes awhile to replace previous poorer choices with newer healthier choices. People will tend to wake up with previous lifestyle stresses ready to reenact, so morning is the best time to immediately start the new habit awareness.

We *don't* count calories or focus on food though some food education is necessary. We don't care if you occasionally eat the "old bad foods" as long as you don't do it every day. The goal is a better overall direction which involves some going back and forth for awhile, so no discouragement of "old you" eating is required, actually it is expected. In fact, when you do eat old patterns you consciously start to experience even more intensely the negative health, mood and energy effects these foods cause or control. Thus you get a very useful "negative" and motivating experience. Then old food eating patterns feel worse, causing less and less frequent return of old food eating drives. I'd rather someone eat 10 candy bars in one day than eat 1 candy bar every day. That is because the negative effects of the occasional bad food will be much more pronounced and conscious to the eater than to someone who eats it every day and thus never experiences normal mood. Once you find enlightened normal mood it is hard to go back to distorted food eating drives and resulting emotions.

All the "Outside" tricks and changes are done to a) gradually change to healthy weight regaining status, and to b) find what is natural for the individual. That allows consciousness and willpower to concern oneself with the true power of emotional living and to be able to affect or manipulate their inner choices and emotional life states to be peaceful, pleasurable and fulfilling - away from need, negativity, depression and reactive living. Gaining the inner thoughts and willpower that help create an emotionally simplified yet heightened, pleasurable you are the permanent curing changes that occur with the *Inside-Outside Diet*.

These changes occur both spontaneously and with directed emotional exercises along the way.

How people respond to losing weight is very individual. For some people, just reading the information in *The Inside Outside Diet* supplies the food and supplement information that they need to regain a better food regimen and therefore weight. For others, simply becoming aware of how they overeat and their personal reasons for overeating empowers them to alter their choices and regain a normal weight. Others have more deeply seated beliefs, drives and emotions that they require a more personal emotional therapy approach to losing weight. This can mean mental and emotional therapy done on an individual basis. In the final analysis, how your personality goes from "reading about" to actualizing the information in this book will be key to your rate of success. Either way, you will be learning more about your weight mechanisms and become more empowered to improve your entire health. The truth is your willpower and conviction to change will be increased as you start to employ all the methods in this book. This happens by increasing your knowledge, distilling your beliefs to positive useful ones and clearing out your emotional clutter with energy stabilizing techniques that do not involve overeating.

Doctor Laursen's first book, *Start Living Stop Dying – 10 Steps to Natural Health*, contains the preliminary work and foundation for everyone's health. *The Inside-Outside Diet* builds upon the principles and information set forth in the former book.

Index of Emotional and Mental Exercises

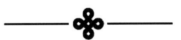

www.NaturalBodyHealth.com